EMERGENCY AND INTENSIVE CARE MEDICINE

# ABDOMINAL TRAUMA AND ABDOMINAL AORTIC ANEURYSMS

## SYMPTOMS, DIAGNOSTIC METHODS AND TREATMENT OUTCOMES

# EMERGENCY AND INTENSIVE CARE MEDICINE

Additional books in this series can be found on Nova's website under the Series tab.

Additional e-books in this series can be found on Nova's website under the e-book tab.

EMERGENCY AND INTENSIVE CARE MEDICINE

# ABDOMINAL TRAUMA AND ABDOMINAL AORTIC ANEURYSMS

## SYMPTOMS, DIAGNOSTIC METHODS AND TREATMENT OUTCOMES

LOUISE SANTIAGO
EDITOR

*New York*

**Library of Congress Cataloging-in-Publication Data**

ISBN: 978-1-63483-482-7

Library of Congress Control Number: 2015946410

*Published by Nova Science Publishers, Inc. † New York*

# CONTENTS

# PREFACE

In this book, the epidemiology, identification of and management of injuries sustained from blunt abdominal trauma (BAT) in childhood are discussed, with a focus on recent advances and future research. Open abdomen (OA), which refers to leaving abdominal incisions open after surgical procedures, and its management are presented as well. Also in this book, bacterial peritonitis and intra-abdominal abscesses, which are major complicated intra-abdominal infections post abdominal trauma are discussed. The severe abdominal consequences of falling, particularly among older adults, is reviewed as well. Finally, periodontitis is known to be a risk factor for abdominal aortic aneurysm (AAA). The authors focus on the role of specific periodontopathic bacteria in AAA and are able to conclude that periodontal pathogens play a major, critical role in AAA development.

Chapter 1 – Fifty years ago, the acceptance of non-operative management of isolated solid organ injuries was a radical advancement in the care of children and youth with blunt abdominal trauma (BAT). Since then, refinements of care of these injury patterns have revolved around protocols for length of bedrest and timing of return to activities, imaging modalities and grading of severity, resuscitation and identification of need for operative intervention or less-invasive arterial embolization, damage-control surgery and techniques to spare loss of the spleen. The concept of regional trauma systems as a means to ensure patients receive definitive treatment at appropriate levels of care has led to further improvements in outcomes with less use of computed tomography (CT) and associated exposure to ionizing radiation and significantly less operative interventions. Ongoing research to identify clinically significant injuries with more judicious use of CT, developing triage guidelines within regional trauma systems, more clearly defining the role of focused abdominal sonography for trauma (FAST) and abbreviating the need of hospital admission for less severe injuries can allow for more efficient use of resources, reduce the impact of prolonged hospitalization on families and the system and optimize outcomes of children and youth with BAT. This chapter will discuss the epidemiology, identification of and management of injuries sustained from BAT in childhood, with a focus on these recent advances and future research.

Chapter 2 – Open abdomen (OA) is a term currently used to refer to leaving abdominal incision open after surgical procedure. Indications for OA management are heterogeneous and consensus has not been reached to date. However, in trauma setting damage control surgery and abdominal compartment syndrome are the most common indications for such treatment. OA is usually managed with temporary abdominal closure (TAC) techniques. TAC is an attempt to control fluid losses, minimize the loss of domain, and to reduce fascial retraction. These techniques are also used as a bridge treatment to facilitate patient management until definitive closure is obtained. OA management is a result of a conjunct effort of surgeons and anesthesiologists. Such collaboration could also increase any possibility to produce high quality evidence in this field: in fact, an agreement about the right timing and method for abdominal closure is still to be obtained. A literature review will be presented to try to clarify crucial aspects of this topic.

Chapter 3 – Bacterial peritonitis and intra-abdominal abscesses are major complicated intra-abdominal infections post abdominal trauma. These infections are often associated with intestinal or mesenteric ischemic injury, hollow organ gangrene or perforation, intra-abdominal visceral laceration, infarction or perforation, severe pancreatitis, penetrating injury and anastomotic fistula. Infections occur following the invasion of pathogenic bacteria into the abdominal cavity or the involved organs. These infections mainly manifest as diffuse peritonitis, peritoneal abscesses, or multiple intra-abdominal visceral abscesses that require treatment combining surgical protocols with anti-infective agents. Sepsis can occur due to the invasion of numerous bacteria and toxins into the blood circulation, which may further progress to septic shock, respiratory distress syndrome, acute renal failure as well as intestinal and hepatic dysfunction.

Currently, the predominant causative bacteria include Gram-negative bacteria, such as *Escherichia coli* (*E. coli*), *Klebsiella pneumoniae (K. pneumoniae*) and *Pseudomonas aeruginosa* (*P. aeruginosa*) as well as Gram-positive bacteria like *Staphylococcus aureus* (*S. aureus*) and *Enterococcus faecalis (E. faecalis).* The widespread multi-drug resistant Gram-negative organisms are challenging physicians to effectively treat these infections.

Followed by the extensive use of broad-spectrum antibiotics, the extended-spectrum β-lactamases (ESBLs) and AmpC β-lactamases have conferred resistance of the Gram-negative organisms to third- and fourth-generation cephalosporins and have limited the choice of antibiotics to carbapenems for therapy against serious infections. As increasing use of carbapenems, however, carbapenem-resistant enterobacteria are alarmingly emerged in the field of trauma-related intra-abdominal infections. Resistance to ertapenem frequently occurs in the ESBL- and/or AmpC-producing enterobacteria with deficiency of outer membrane porin genes, such as loss or truncated mutation of *ompK35* and *ompK36* in *K. pneumoniae.* Whereas resistances to imipenem and/or meropenem usually necessity additional production of carbapenemases, such as *K. pneumoniae* carbapenemase (KPC) and New Delhi metallo-β-lactamase 1 (NDM-1).

Amikacin, gentamicin, fosfomycin, tigecycline and colistin are active versus most isolates of the KPC-producing enterobacteria, whereas only tigecycline and colistin remain active versus most NDM-1 isolates. Vancomycin and teicoplanin remain active against *S. aureus* isolates. Fosfomycin, tigecycline, daptomycin and linezolid are potential candidates to treat most Gram-positive bacteria, especially with vancomycin resistance.

In summary, surgical source control and combination therapies with the most potent anti-infective agents are indicated to treat the patients with trauma-related intra-abdominal serious infections, based on the local bacterial susceptibility epidemiology.

Chapter 4 – Elderly community-dwelling patients often experience ground-level falls: one out of three adults aged 65 and older falls each year and the incidence increases to 50% in those over 80 years old. Following a fall, the patient is usually brought to the emergency department where fractures or brain injury are the major concern and serious abdominal injury is seldom contemplated.

We used a retrospective chart analysis to identify all such patients presenting after a simple fall and admitted with serious blunt abdominal trauma to a single academic medical centre. Out of 546 patients screened, 3 cases of ground-level falls leading to splenic rupture; isolated gallbladder rupture with gallstone ileus; and perinephric hematoma were found (0.55%) and are reported. The literature on other serious abdominal consequences of falls and non-penetrating 'minor' abdominal trauma among older adults not encountered in our series was reviewed to capture the whole spectrum of abdominal adverse events of falls in elderly patients. In conclusion, Falls in elderly patients are exceedingly common mandating recognition of even rare complications. Physicians should be more aware of the possibility of occult and serious consequences of blunt abdominal trauma after falls among older adults, albeit rare.

Chapter 5 - Periodontitis is known to be a risk factor for abdominal aortic aneurysm (AAA). However, the influence of periodontitis on AAA development is to be elucidated. The aim of this article was to review the relationship between periodontal bacterial burden and AAA. We focused on the roles of specific periodontopathic bacteria in AAA, matrix metalloproteinases and toll-like receptors in the pathophysiology in the section of experimental analysis. Furthermore, we showed clinical data of periodontitis in patients with AAA and other cardiovascular diseases. We concluded that periodontal pathogens play a critical role in the AAA development.

In: Abdominal Trauma ...
Editor: Louise Santiago
ISBN: 978-1-63483-482-7


***Chapter 1***

# BLUNT ABDOMINAL TRAUMA IN CHILDREN

***Natalie L. Yanchar, MD, MSc, FRCSC***
Associate Professor in Surgery, Emergency Medicine and Community Health and Epidemiology, Dalhousie University
Halifax, Nova Scotia, Canada

## ABSTRACT

Fifty years ago, the acceptance of non-operative management of isolated solid organ injuries was a radical advancement in the care of children and youth with blunt abdominal trauma (BAT). Since then, refinements of care of these injury patterns have revolved around protocols for length of bedrest and timing of return to activities, imaging modalities and grading of severity, resuscitation and identification of need for operative intervention or less-invasive arterial embolization, damage-control surgery and techniques to spare loss of the spleen. The concept of regional trauma systems as a means to ensure patients receive definitive treatment at appropriate levels of care has led to further improvements in outcomes with less use of computed tomography (CT) and associated exposure to ionizing radiation and significantly less operative interventions. Ongoing research to identify clinically significant injuries with more judicious use of CT, developing triage guidelines within regional trauma systems, more clearly defining the role of focused abdominal sonography for trauma (FAST) and abbreviating the need of hospital admission for less severe injuries can allow for more efficient use of resources, reduce the impact of prolonged hospitalization on families and the system and optimize outcomes of children and youth with BAT. This chapter will discuss the epidemiology, identification of and management of injuries sustained from BAT in childhood, with a focus on these recent advances and future research.

## INTRODUCTION

It is well known that injuries kill more children in the developed world than all other diseases combined [1]. In the developing world, injuries rank second to communicable diseases as the leading cause of pediatric deaths [1-3]. Road traffic accidents, frequently associated with significant trunkal trauma, is heralded by the WHO as one of the emerging diseases to affect children [4].

After traumatic brain injuries, abdominal trauma ranks as the second most common injury type to be related to mortality from injury in the pediatric population. Although there are areas of the world, both in North American and other continents, where violence and penetrating injuries are a reality for many children, for the most part abdominal trauma in children results from blunt mechanisms.

Dependent on the age of the child, mechanisms of injury resulting in BAT can vary significantly. Toddlers tend to be involved in more "situational" traumatic events, including motor vehicle crashes, pedestrian, falls from open windows and falls in playgrounds. Older children tend to be involved in mechanisms/situations associated with risk-taking, whether it be a bicycling, pedestrian, motor vehicle crashes, motor vehicle crashes or flipping on all-terrain vehicles.

Anatomic differences from adults make children more prone to intraabdominal injuries with blunt forces. The more horizontal lie of the diaphragm and the shallowness of the pelvis leaves upper abdominal organs and pelvic organs (especially the bladder) less protected by the rib cage and pelvic bones, respectively.

The thinner, less muscular abdominal wall is less protective, and compared to adults, there is far less intraabdominal and retroperitoneal cushioning fat, leaving the intraabdominal organs more prone to impact from direct blows or compression against the vertebral column (as with a bicycle handlebar or lap belt injury mechanism).

## Mechanisms of Intraabdominal Injuries in Children

There are several common patterns of injuries that can occur in children dependent upon the mechanism. These include lapbelt injuries during motor vehicle crashes, pedestrian injuries, direct blows to the abdomen, most notable seen with bicycle handlebars and non-accidental trauma [5, 6].

Motor vehicle crashes associated with use of lap belts are one of the most common mechanisms of trauma resulting in significant pediatric intraabdominal injuries. These typically result from a frontal car crash with children who are too small for a seat belt alone, restrained by a lap belt only – either in an older vehicle with only lap belts or having placed the shoulder portion of a three point restraint behind them [7]. Acting as a fulcrum, the belt creates an acute compression across the mid to upper abdomen, riding upwards as the child ‘submarines’ under it. The typical triad of injuries with this mechanism includes an abdominal wall contusion following the course of the lap belt, intraabdominal injuries and a distraction injury of the spine – either a Chance fracture alone or combined with a spinal cord injury.

Suspicion of an intraabdominal injury should always be considered with this mechanism of injury. A review of several case series by Achildi et al. suggests that up to 75% of children presenting with abdominal wall ecchymoses may have a significant intraabdominal injury [8]. A recent prospective study by the Pediatric Emergency Care Applied Research Network (PECARN) found this number to be 19%, although this maybe falsely lowered due to more selective use of CT scanning in their study population [9]. Typical intraabdominal injuries with this mechanism include solid organ contusions or lacerations and small bowel hematomas, perforations or transections [10]. Injuries to the mesentery can also occur which may or may not result in clinically significant sequelae [7, 11, 12]. If intestinal devascularization occurs, ischemia may progress to necrosis and delayed perforation over hours to days, or even later evolve into an ischemic stricture or intestinal fistula [13, 14]. Less commonly, a retroperitoneal injury can occur, the potentially most devastating being to the aorta being an aortic injury [15, 16]. Imaging, usually with CT and intravenous contrast, is needed in most cases of lap belt injuries if the child is hemodynamically stable.

A history of direct impact with the end of a bicycle handlebar should also raise suspicion of an injury. Typically, the child hits an object while riding their bicycle, acutely turning the handle bar sideways while falling forward into it. In classic cases, the round imprint of the handlebar may be seen on the abdominal wall. Compression in the upper midline across the vertebral column typically results in liver, pancreatic and/or duodenal injuries, although other sites of injury can also be seen [17-20]. Depending on the force of impact, initial clinical signs and symptoms may be subtle and careful monitoring is required because of risk of later-presenting ischemic injuries [17].

Intraabdominal injuries in toddlers, and especially infants, should always heighten awareness of the risk of nonaccidental trauma (NAT). A review of childhood hospitalizations in the US recently demonstrated that up to 25% of children <12 months of age admitted within intraabdominal injuries were the result of NAT [6, 21]. Duodenal injuries in particular are commonly a result of physical abuse (from a blow to the abdomen) and abuse should always be considered when a duodenal injury is encountered in a young patient. One multicenter review reported that 100% of duodenal injuries in children under age 2 years and 54% in children 3–5 years old were as a result of child abuse [22]. Similarly, Gaines et al, of 30 patients with duodenal injuries in their series, all eight of those under the age of 4 resulted from NAT [23].

## Initial Management

Initial management of any pediatric patient must be predicated on ensuring stabilization of the cardiorespiratory status. Assessment and protection of the ABC's ("Airway, Breathing and Circulation") represents the primary assessment of the patient, with a head-to-toe evaluation of all body systems comprising the secondary survey. Dependent on the situation, a urinary catheter to decompress the bladder and nasogastric (NG) tube to decompress the stomach may be of great use for the further assessment. The younger and more frightened the child, the more crying and air swallowing they will do. This can result in significant gastric distention which can make clinical assessment of the abdomen more difficult. In the hemodynamically unstable patient, with tachycardia, with or without hypotension to suggest hypovolemia, the source of blood loss must be identified and quickly. Common sites of acute blood loss in children include intraabdominal organs (solid and vascular), femur fractures, hemothoraces and highly vascularized soft tissue injuries such as scalp lacerations.

The goal of resuscitation is to establish cardiorespiratory stability to provide time to diagnose and manage specific injuries. Classically, this involves infusion of isotonic crystalloid such as normal saline with a 20cc/kg bolus. This should be repeated as needed; however, little response to the first bolus should prompt emergent access to blood products, with delivery of packed red blood cells (typically 10 cc/kg boluses with repeats as needed) with infusion initiated if there is little to no response to infusion of a second bolus of crystalloid, or earlier. In the child who remains unstable, emergent identification of the likely sources of blood loss must be made. Splinting of femur fractures, wrapping the pelvis in a bed sheet or specific pelvic binder and pressure on actively bleeding soft tissue wounds may control ongoing hemorrhage from these sites. Although nonoperative management of most solid organ injuries in children can be successful, even those that appear catastrophic on imaging, for persistent hemodynamic instability with no other obvious bleeding source an urgent laparotomy may be the only means of vascular control. The role of FAST to confirm hemoperitoneum in the unstable child is still not well defined [24] and local expertise in point of care USS may dictate its use. However, in the unstable child, the presence of free intraperitoneal fluid in such an instance may expedite the decision to proceed with laparotomy. Regardless, the clinical status of the child should take precedence and unwarranted delays to definitive hemodynamic control, resulting from imaging to look for free fluid, must be avoided.

## Diagnosis

There has been much literature published to determine tools to aid the clinician in definitive diagnoses and subsequent management of blunt abdominal injuries in children. These are predicated on clinical signs and symptoms, specific laboratory values and imaging. It is important to note that no one "rule" will fit every situation. Decisions will depend on local resources and expertise, comfort levels of the clinical team with the various ages and stages of infants to adolescents, and triage and transfer protocols or guidelines of the local-regional trauma system. Undoubtedly, approach to the injured child will vary depending on if the child has arrived at a rural hospital with limited resources versus a Level I Pediatric Trauma Centre. It is of infinite value for all clinical institutions within a defined trauma system to have well-established guidelines of what patients are best served with transfer to a higher level of care for definitive diagnoses and management versus definitive care at the local level, which has the advantage of keeping children and families closer to their communities and not overwhelming the regional pediatric trauma centre with lesser acuity patients.

## Clinical Features

As described above, the injured child with hemodynamic instability that cannot be attributed to another source than then abdomen may not provide enough time for laboratory studies or imaging before definitive surgical control is needed. For these cases or those who have achieved stability with initial resuscitation, signs such as abdominal distention, abdominal wall bruising, and tenderness or guarding to palpation are strongly associated with the presence of intraabdominal injuries [5, 25]. The sensitivity and specificity of these findings significantly diminish with decreasing levels of consciousness and may not be reliable in those with a decreased Glasgow Coma Score (GCS) [26].

In large reported series of children with BAT, it is not unusual to have a small proportion of cases who present with none to minimal clinical signs or symptoms of intraabdominal injury, yet ultimately become diagnosed with a significant injuries, often of hollow viscus organs [9, 13]. Initial CT findings in these patients may show no evidence of free air, but may demonstrate nonspecific findings such as free fluid or mesenteric stranding. Many believe that repeat physical examination of these patients is warranted to recognize a delayed presentation of a hollow viscus injury, the most common being of the small intestine. Whether such presentation is due to a "missed" diagnosis or due to delay in development as ischemia proceeds to necrosis and then perforation may be debated, but regardless, highlights the well-described tenet that the best way to identify intestinal injuries is with serial examination [13, 14].

Mechanism of trauma, as described above, in association with clinical signs and symptoms may also suggest presence or absence of injuries that require further investigation. To the fact, after review of a large series of children 4 years and older with BAT, subsequently diagnosed with liver or spleen injuries, Acker et al. found that in the context of a low risk, single non-motorized mechanism (e.g., falls, sports) and low risk clinical criteria (normal GCS, normal age-adjusted ratio of heart rate/systolic blood pressure), none of the 101 children meeting these low risk criteria required any interventions [27]. They concluded that it may be possible to manage patients with such low-risk features with a short period of observation in the ED, with discharge instruction of some activity restrictions, without definitive diagnosis by CT. Further work is needed to develop an evidence-informed observation algorithm for such patients.

## Laboratory Studies

The utility of laboratory studies is often questioned in the acute work-up of a child with possible intraabdominal injuries. Capraro et al. demonstrated the sensitivity and specificity of identifying an abdominal injury (confirmed by CT) of elevated serum levels of aspartate aminotransferase (AST) to be 63% and 48% respectively, of serum amylase to be 6% and 95%, respectively, and of hematuria on urinalysis to be 52% and 50%, respectively [28]. Because of the low sensitivities and positive predictive values in their patient population, they suggest that routine "trauma panel" blood work should not be undertaken in all trauma patients. Hynick et al. demonstrated in their patient population, an elevated serum alanine aminotransferase (ALT) was independently associated with a 4-fold increase risk of identifying an intraabdominal injury on CT [5]. However, when only clinically significant injuries were considered (grade III or higher of solid organ injuries or any hollow-viscus injury), it was no longer significant [5]. Hematuria (gross or microscopic), however, remained significantly associated when controlling for other predictive variables [5]. This has also been described by others [25].

In isolation, laboratory values are unlikely to be useful in predicting injuries. However, in combination with physical findings and initial screening imaging, they have been proven useful in helping to triage patients for more definitive imaging and/or to higher levels of care [29]. (See *Decision-Support Tools*, below).

## FAST

The use of Focused Abdominal Sonography for Trauma (FAST) initially evolved to replace peritoneal lavage for assessment of the hemodynamically unstable trauma patient in whom rapid identification of free fluid in the peritoneal cavity would indicate an abdominal source of bleeding and rapidly triage the patient to the operating room for definitive control of bleeding. Its use in the pediatric population, however, is still unclear, especially since most children with even significant bleeding from solid organ injuries, stabilize with resuscitative measures and can successfully undergo nonoperative management of their injuries. As with the adult population, FAST focuses on detecting free intraperitoneal fluid within any of the right upper quadrant hepatorenal recess (Morrison's pouch), the left upper quadrant perisplenic view, the upper midline subxiphoid window to examine the pericardial sac fluid signifying cardiac tamponade, and the suprapubic window to look for free fluid in the pelvis (Pouch of Dougla)s. An extended or "E-FAST" can be done that also examines both hemithoraces to look for hemo- and/or pneumothoraces.

During assessment in the acute phase of trauma care, CT scanning remains the gold standard for identifying intraabdominal injuries, yet comes with a significant risk of radiation exposure to children. As such, researchers have looked at ways in which FAST can be used to screen or triage children with BAT to need for CT scanning. Menaker and the PECARN group, studying the use of FAST across pediatric emergency departments in the US, found increased use with increasing suspicion of the presence of an intraabdominal injury [24]. Moreover, they observed decreased use of abdominal CT scanning of patients in whom the suspicion of an injury was low to moderate and who received a FAST exam, suggesting that a negative exam can add to the assessing physician's comfort level in ruling out a clinically significant injury without the use of more definitive imaging [24].

A metanalysis of FAST exams in children by Holmes et al. demonstrated a moderate sensitivity (66%) but high specificity (95%) in detecting intraperitoneal fluid [30]. Thus, if free fluid is seen, it may be necessary to pursue further imaging to more clearly delineate what injuries are present. Contrarily, a negative FAST examination has generally poor utility as a means to rule out intraabdominal injuries when used alone. However, as shown by Menaker and others, it can be of potential use when suspicion of an intraabdominal injury is already present [30]. Further work is required to determine the role of FAST in the assessment and diagnosis of intraabdominal injuries in children with BAT.

## Decision-Support Tools

Much work has been done in the last several years to develop decision-support tools to aid the clinician in deciding the need for definitive cross-sectional imaging with CT scanning as a means to reduce the risk of radiation to the pediatric patient while not risking missing clinically significant intraabdominal injuries. In 2002, Holmes and colleagues prospectively studied children assessed in the emergency department for blunt torso trauma and determined 6 features that were associated with ultimately identifying an intraabdominal injury on CT scan: low systolic blood pressure, abdominal tenderness, femur fracture, elevated liver tranasaminases, urinalysis with more than 5 red blood cells per high-powered field and an initial hematocrit of less than 30% [31]. Prospectively studied, the absence of any or all of these variables was able to predict the lack of an intraabdominal injury in another large cohort, with a false negative rate of only 2% [25]. Similar findings were demonstrated by Hynick et al. with abdominal tenderness, hematuria and elevated serum ALT being independently predictive of clinically significant intraabdominal injury [5]. A subsequent study by the PECARN group has shown that absence of seven clinical findings in patients presenting to the ED (evidence of abdominal wall trauma or seat belt sign, Glasgow Coma Scale score less than 14, abdominal tenderness, evidence of thoracic wall trauma, complaints of abdominal pain, decreased breath sounds, and vomiting) can safely rule out the presence of any clinically significant intraabdominal injuries in over 99% of patients without need for CT imaging [32]. Contrarily, however, its high sensitivity but very low specificity in identifying patients in need of imaging to identify clinically important injuries (99% and 56%, respectively) suggests that the addition of laboratory and/or FAST exams may increase the specificity to make such decision support tools of greater clinical utility [32].

## Definitive Imaging

Imaging modalities available to the clinician include plain radiographs, ultrasound (whether point of care or "FAST" or detailed sonography), computed tomography and magnetic resonance imaging (MRI). Choice of modality will depend on expertise available, degree of suspicion of the presence of an intraabdominal injury, how clinically significant that injury may be and how the results will influence management. Dependent on triage protocols of the regional trauma system, imaging may be deferred until transfer to definitive care so as to reduce delays in transfer and reduce unnecessary or duplicate imaging.

Suspicion of a perforated viscus (either by mechanism or clinical signs of peritonitis) mandates a plain radiograph. Free air on a cross-table lateral view, or if the patient is able to log roll, above the liver on a right lateral decubitus view, is pathognomonic of a perforated viscus in this scenario, and mandates laparotomy or laparoscopy. Whether or not cross sectional imaging with CT is required pre-operatively will depend on the clinician's suspicion of a concomitant solid organ, retroperitoneal or other injury and whether such pre-operative knowledge would change acute operative management.

Ultrasound has the advantage of being able to determine the presence of free intraperitoneal fluid and look at specific organs, especially solid organs, without concerns of ionizing radiation. Its disadvantages include lack of ability to delineate solid organ injuries in the early phases of trauma, variability depending on the patient body habitus, especially obese patients, and strong dependency on operator expertise [30]. As such, it is rarely used for the definitive diagnoses of intraabdominal injuries, especially in North America. It has, however, been more favored in European countries for assessment of blunt trauma in all ages. More recently, the development of contrast-enhanced ultrasound (CEUS) has significantly improved the utility of ultrasound in the acute assessment of trauma patients [33]. Injection of microbubbles which stay in the vascular system allows clearer definition of solid tissues, pooling of blood and in many instances images almost as clear as those from CT scanning. Limitations include inability to visualize extravasation from the renal collecting system (as the microbubbles disappear once extravasated) as well as the technical limitations of conventional ultrasound listed above [33]. Recent publications from Europe indicate that this modality is almost as sensitive and specific for solid organ injuries as conventional CT scanning when assessing blunt torso trauma in children. Further studies on its use in pediatric trauma are needed before more generalized acceptance is taken up [34].

Until then, the gold standard for imaging of blunt pediatric imaging remains CT scanning. Undoubtedly, visualization of extent/degree of solid organ injuries, visualization of the retroperitoneum and findings such as mesenteric streaking or free fluid without definitive solid organ hemorrhage to suggest an intestinal or bladder injury, is clearer with CT than ultrasound. On the other hand, a completely unremarkable CT is over 99% predictive of the absence of an intraabdominal injury and, in the context of the entire clinical and social picture, could be used to justify discharge from the emergency department of an otherwise stable child with no other overt injuries [35].

The major disadvantage of CT scanning in the pediatric population is the high levels of radiation doses delivered to the patient. Work by Brenner et al, modeling from the radiation-induced cancer risk of nuclear bomb victims, estimated that of the annual 600,000 abdominal and head CT examinations performed on U.S. children less than 15 years old in 1999, approximately 500 would ultimately die from a cancer attributable to the radiation from the CT [36]. More recent work by Miglioretti et al. using US data from 1996 to 2010 estimated that approximately 4870 future cancers would be attributed to pediatric CT scanning each year in the US [37]. More importantly however, was that reducing the highest 25% of doses within age groups and anatomic regions to the median dose could prevent 43% of these cancers, reducing the number of exams performed by 33% could reduce the number of future cancers by one third and that combining the 2 approaches could prevent 62% of these cancers overall [37]. It must be noted that many of these large epidemiologic modeling studies have been challenged in the context of educating physicians on the value of CT scans that are clinically justified, such that their benefit far outweighs their estimated risk [38]. Regardless, the "ALARA" (As Low As Reasonably Achievable) principle, promoted by the Alliance For Radiation Safety in Pediatric Imaging and referring to the amount of radiation required to achieve high quality imaging that provides the information needed in the best interest of the patient , should always be considered when imaging a child with CT. Efforts should be made to use pediatric radiation doses, sharing of images between referring centers to avoid repeat scanning, selectively scanning only those body regions of need and whenever possible, choosing imaging modalities that can provide equivalent information at lower radiation costs [39].

## Definitive Management

Management of intraabdominal injuries in children, as in adults, is dependent upon many factors including type, degree, presence and type of other injuries, age of the child and presence of comorbidities, and clinical and physical resources available. Ideally, triage and transfer of inured children should occur so that optimal outcomes can be attained with the most cost effective and efficient use of resources. Clearly, not all injured children require definitive treatment in a designated pediatric trauma centre, including not all of those with intraabdominal injuries. Lack of hemodynamic stability will dictate the need for definitive surgical control using resources available to the site of initial triage. Whether this can be dealt with pressure or other simple maneuvers to stop hemorrhage or requires packing and other damage-control maneuvers with rapid transfer to critical care to control hypothermia, sepsis and coagulopathy, will be case-dependent. Stable patients may or may not require transfer, dependent upon the factors outlined above. In these cases, ideally, predetermined lines of communication have already been established between the regional pediatric trauma centre and the referral hospitals to provide advice and establish transfer agreements and guidelines predicated on the best practices of management for these patients and their families.

## Intestinal Injuries

Clear visualization of pneumoperitoneum on pain radiographs or CT in the setting of BAT represents a hollow viscus injury in need of operative attention. In many cases, however, imaging may not be as overtly obvious upon initial presentation of the child. It is important to look for indirect signs of mesenteric or bowel wall trauma that may ultimately progress to loss of intestinal integrity due to latent ischemia. A recent review by Khasawneh et al. list several findings on CT, some of which can be fairly subtle, that could be associated with intestinal injury including free fluid in the absence of solid organ injury, absent or enhanced bowel wall enhancement, mesenteric hematoma, active mesenteric extravasation of intravenous contrast and mesenteric stranding [40]. Although these findings can be seen in isolation with an intestinal injury, they are more diagnostic when seen in combination and careful review of the scans in the setting of potential intestinal injury is mandatory. Regardless, if intestinal injury is not initially obvious, serial examination and assessment of the patient is crucial as ischemia may progress to delayed perforation. It is also important to recognize that ischemia or direct bowel injury may also progress to scarring and ultimately an intestinal stricture and obstruction due to stricture several weeks later. Walled-off perforations have also been reported to present in this way [14]. For children followed with non-operative management of BAT, post-discharge advice to be aware of development of obstructive symptoms should be given].

As discussed above, intestinal injuries may not be evident, even to the most astute physician, at the time of initial presentation and work-up, but may be suspected based on mechanism or initial imaging. Strong clinical acumen to understand the risk of an intestinal injury requiring surgical management requires repeat examination and assessment of the child over time. Some have advocated for early laparotomy/laparoscopy in cases where suspicion of injury is very high, such as in cases of lap belt mechanisms [41]. However, close monitoring and repeat assessments are well-accepted, also providing opportunity to transfer to higher levels of care should that be required. If intervened upon later, when clinically evident, yet within the first 24 hours after presentation to the ED, outcomes are unlikely to be worse than if diagnosed promptly upon first assessment [42]. More prolonged delay can be associated with significant morbidity due to sepsis [43]. Close observation and reassessment of children with blunt trauma, at risk for intestinal injury, is imperative [13, 43].

Once an intestinal injury is diagnosed, surgery should not be delayed so as to reduce the risk of development of sepsis. In a hemodynamically stable child, whether repair is approached laparoscopically or with laparotomy depends upon the surgical skills and resources of the provider. Indeed, laparoscopy has been demonstrated to be equally effective in repair of intestinal injuries [44]. In most cases, simple repair or resection with primary anastomosis may be all that is required. Need for ostomies or simply stapling off the bowel to rapidly remove devitalized segments in cases of concern for healing or in cases of massive peritoneal soiling or damage control surgery in an unstable patient remains a "safe" approach [45]. However, with good intraoperative peritoneal lavage and perioperative monitoring, including adequate nutrition, primary anastomoses, even with colonic injuries, can be successful.

## Spleen & Liver

The management of solid organ injuries in children, especially the spleen, has evolved significantly over the past four decades. Splenectomy was traditionally the standard of care for traumatic splenic injuries up until the 1970's [46]. In 1968, Upadhyaya and Simpson published one of the first series of nonoperative management of splenic injuries in children, concluding it to be a viable management option in the stable child with no other reason for laparotomy [47]. Since then, with the recognition that operative intervention creates risks of morbidity associated with a large abdominal incision, prolonged course of recovery and surgical risks of uncontrollable intraoperative hemorrhage with ensuing coagulopathy [41], non-operative management has become the standard of care for hemodynamically stable children with blunt splenic and/or liver trauma, successful in over 95% of cases [24, 48-50]. Compared to operative intervention, it is associated with significant reduction in need for critical care services, overall hospital stay, use of follow up imaging, length of activity restriction, long-term complications and is overall more cost-effective [51-53]. More importantly, it avoids surgical risks and infection by encapsulated organisms in the form of post-splenectomy sepsis [54].

In the case of a hemodynamically unstable child who is found at laparotomy to have a splenic injury as the cause of bleeding, splenectomy is the most expeditious surgical option for vascular control. Dependent upon the status of the child and the skill of the surgeon, other surgical options include splenorrhaphy using large dissolvable sutures or wrapping of the spleen in a biodegradable mesh [55, 56]. For those who are initially deemed to be stable enough for observation, but then become unstable despite blood transfusions, angiography with embolization is an option if available. The success of angiography is suggested by a trend noted by Lee at al using the Kids' Inpatient Database in the US [57]. Between 2000 and 2008, there was a significant decline in splenectomy rates for children from splenic trauma, associated with a significant increase in angiography and embolization rates (from 2.4% to 6.9%) [57]. How much of the decision to proceed with this intervention is based on true need versus physician comfort level with nonoperative management without embolization is not clear however. Li et al. comparing non-pediatric to pediatric general surgeons showed that the former would be twice as likely to intervene with embolization in face of a contrast blush on CT as the latter [58]. Even more, others are reporting that with careful management of splenic injuries in dedicated pediatric hospitals, these can be successfully managed with no intervention at all aside from careful observation in over 95% of pediatric patients.

In the hemodynamically stable child with a splenic or liver injury, it has become clear from the literature that severity of injury, as measured by CT grading, is not an indicator of need for intervention. Yang et al. presented a series of grade IV and V spleen and liver injuries, all successfully managed non-operatively without significant complications [59]. Fremgen et al. similarly demonstrated that physiologic criteria, alone, are sufficient to predict need for laparotomy the case of major pediatric liver trauma [60]. As indicated above, active extravasation of intravenous contrast seen on CT (contrast "blush") is considered by some to be an indicator for need of splenic artery embolization [61]. Others, however, have found no association between the presence of a contrast blush and short or long-term complications with nonoperative management without embolization [62-64]. Davies et al. found that of 123 patients with blunt splenic injuries at their institution, seven percent had a blush seen on CT scan, which was associated with low hemoglobin levels and laboratory evidence of some ongoing bleeding but was not associated with need for transfusion, prolonged length of stay mortality or need for operative intervention [62]. The use of angiography with embolization for blunt liver trauma in children has also been reported, especially in those who require ongoing fluid and blood resuscitation and have a blush seen on CT [65, 66]. Ultimately, adjuncts to non-operative treatment of these solid-organ injuries is dependent on the clinical status of the patient, the expertise and resources available and comfort level of the clinical team caring for the child.

To promote the use of nonoperative management of blunt splenic injuries, the American Pediatric Surgical Association has developed guidelines, which have been prospectively evaluated for the management of these patients based on CT grade, and are presented in Table 1 [51, 67]. Since then, a further abbreviated bedrest protocol has been evaluated by St. Peter et al. and shown to be equally as safe as these guidelines while further limiting the use of hospital resources [68].

**Table 1. American Pediatric Surgical Association: Guidelines for Resource Utilization in Children with Isolated Spleen or Liver Injury [67]**

| | CT Grade | | | |
|---|---|---|---|---|
| | I | II | III | IV |
| ICU days | None | None | None | 1 |
| Hospital Stay | 2 | 3 | 4 | 5 |
| Predischarge imaging | None | None | None | None |
| Postdischarge imaging | None | None | None | None |
| Activity restriction (wk)* | 3 | 4 | 5 | 6 |

*Return to full-contact, competitive sports (i.e., football, wrestling, hockey, lacrosse, mountain climbing) should be at the discretion of the individual pediatric trauma surgeon. The proposed guidelines for return to unrestricted activity include "normal" age-appropriate activities.

Despite the demonstrated benefits of nonoperative management with publication of strong guidelines, many physicians do not adhere to guidelines and continue to manage blunt spleen injury operatively. This leads to significant variation in the treatment of pediatric patients with traumatic splenic injuries, especially between centres with pediatric trauma expertise and those without. In fact, several studies have demonstrated a significantly increased risk of splenectomy for blunt splenic trauma in children in non-pediatric centres versus pediatric trauma centres [50, 69-72].This may be due to the general lesser comfort with managing these children without an intervention, by non-pediatric specialists versus by those comfortable with pediatric trauma [58, 73, 74]. In addition to disseminating guidelines for management [72], it is important that triage and transfer policies are established within geographic trauma systems to ensure that all pediatric trauma patients with these and other injuries are ultimately managed where the most optimal outcomes can be ensured [48, 74].

## Pancreatic Injuries

Injuries to the pancreas are not common in children. Fewer than 10% of children sustaining BAT will have pancreatic injury, yet suspicion of its' potential must always be considered in those sustaining direct trauma to the epigastrium (bicycle handlebar injuries, hockey stick injuries, non-accidental trauma) and those with significant energy transfer to the abdomen with blunt impact (pedestrian trauma, motor vehicle occupant injuries and nonaccidental trauma) [18, 75, 76]. Compression of the pancreas against the spine to which it is directly juxtaposed leads to its typical injury pattern in the mid-body. With its retroperitoneal location, it may not be clinically distinct from the presentation of other abdominal injuries (complaints of pain, abdominal tenderness) and later, nausea and vomiting [77, 78]. Elevations in serum amylase and/or lipase are often present, but individually, are not highly sensitive or specific for diagnosis, particularly within the first 3-6 hours post injury [78, 79]. When elevated, several recent studies have shown them to be nonspecific for prediction of need for surgery or development of complications for already identified pancreatic injuries, questioning the need for routine repeat values after initial clinical presentation [79-81]. Others, however, have demonstrated that persistent elevation or ongoing increase of serum amylase and/or lipase may indicate the presence of a yet unidentified pancreatic injury not yet diagnoses by standard imaging [79].

With generally non-specific presentation of clinical signs, symptoms and laboratory values, clinical diagnosis of pancreatic injury in children is challenging. Reliability of the CT scan appears to be less in the first 24 hours after the injury owing to minimal early reactive edema and the relative lack of retroperitoneal fat planes in children [82]. Definitive signs of the presence of a pancreatic injury include injury to the substance of the gland itself: active pancreatic bleeding, pancreatic hematoma, laceration or focal or diffuse enlargement or edema of the gland [83]. Ductal injuries, in particular, can be easily missed on CT. Nonetheless, definitive imaging is required when suspected, particularly with definition of disruption of the, main pancreatic duct, from which ongoing leak of pancreatic enzymes lead to late term sequelae including pancreatitis and development of a pseudocyst.

In a recent review by Potoka et al. it would appear that the sensitivity and specificity of CT in identifying pancreatic injuries ranges from 47 to- 60% [84]. Identification of an actual ductal injury was also relatively low, ranging from 52 to 54% with a specificity of 90% [84]. This underscores the difficulty in making these diagnoses early in the post-injury period, suggesting the need for other modalities should pancreatic injury still be suspected, including both magnetic resonance cholangiopancreatography (MRCP) and/or magnetic endoscopic retrograde cholangiopancreatography (ERCP). A recent study by Garvey et al. demonstrated the utility of ERCP in not only identifying distinct ductal injuries in children, but also its role in treatment. As an adjunct to non-operative management, placement of a therapeutic stent across the ductal disruption, with or without a sphincterotomy may promote normal drainage in patients as young as 5 years of age [85]. MRCP has also been successfully used to more clearly delineate the presence of a pancreatic injury not seen on CT, including the presence of ductal injuries, although it has no direct therapeutic roles [82].

One of the greatest and still-lingering controversies in the management of blunt pancreatic trauma in children is the management of those cases where there is a definitive ductal injury. Using the classification of pancreatic injures, as defined by the American Association of Surgery for Trauma (AAST), grades I and II involve only parenchymal trauma while grades III-V involve the pancreatic duct [83]. Non-operative management of grades I and II injuries is fairly well-accepted. Bowel rest with NG drainage and parenteral nutrition remains the mainstay of treatment. Serial physical examinations and monitoring of serum amylase can be used to judge improvement; their normalization being signs of when to start introduction of oral nutrition again.

For those injuries with ductal disruption, many centres utilize non-operative management, as described above, recognizing that the majority (35-100% in recent series) will ultimately go onto development of a pancreatic pseudocyst [86-91]. Management of the pseudocyst can generally be done successfully with minimally invasive methods, either by percutaneous drainage or endoscopic-placed cyst-gastrostomy stents [82, 90, 91]. Recently Houben et al. have demonstrated the benefit of stent placement by ERCP in not only promoting drainage, but also significantly reducing the risk of pseudocyst development [82].

Many centres advocate for surgical intervention in cases of defined ductal injury, with early operative control with a spleen-saving distal pancreatectomy. Improvements in minimally invasive techniques and experience permit this to be done laparoscopically in an increasing proportion of patients [92]. Complications of surgical intervention are recognized, including bleeding, pancreatic leaks and persistent pancreatic fistulae and inadvertent splenectomy [82]. Despite this, there is undoubtedly an advantage in terms of decreased length of stay and need for parenteral nutrition in patients undergoing early surgical intervention. Iqbal et al. demonstrated in a larger series of children with grade III or greater pancreatic injuries, the time to goal feeds during admission was decreased by 3-fold in those undergoing early operative management (9 versus 26 days) and total days in hospital were significantly reduced (12.5 versus 17.5). Because of a considerable number of children requiring readmission in the nonoperative management group, there was a significant 4-fold increase in total time to resolution in the nonoperative group (19 versus 82 days) [87]. Beres et al. published similar findings [88]. They also reported a significantly higher complication rate of 74% with nonoperative management versus 27% in those undergoing surgery [88]. However, if the development of pseudocysts, which may resolve on their own or be managed with minimally invasive techniques, was excluded from their list of complications, the overall complication rates appeared to be similar between two approaches [88]. Overall, there exists a high degree of complexity and controversy in the literature about how to optimally manage children with pancreatic injury. A systematic review of the literature found that in general, good results are achieved with nonoperative management, but prospective trials are needed in order to adequately evaluate these methods [93].

Ultimately, management of pancreatic injuries is dependent upon the status of the child, the presence of other associated injuries that may require operative intervention (such as a concomitant duodenal injury) and the resources and expertise of the clinical team. Because of the complex nature of these injuries, triage and transfer to definitive care to the regional centre with expertise in pediatric trauma care is recommended.

## Renal Injuries

As with intraabdominal organs, those in the retroperitoneum, most specifically the kidney, are more susceptible to injury in children with blunt trauma than in adults, and more easily sustain more severe injuries [94]. This is likely related to the relative increased size and mobility of the kidney in addition to relatively less protection due to underdevelopment of the flank muscles, more cartilaginous and thus pliable nature of the rib cage and less cushioning by perirenal fat [94]. Frank genitourinary (GU) injuries in blunt trauma are relatively uncommon in children, being found in only 1.5% of children with BAT in one large series [95]. Conversely, hematuria, especially microscopic, is common with BAT of significant force to sustain intraabdominal injuries that may not include visible GU injuries on cross sectional imaging, as noted above [5, 94]. Of 299 pediatric patents with BAT undergoing urinalysis upon presentation, 22% had microscopic hematuria; half of these had clinical findings warranting imaging with CT and of these 91% demonstrated no obvious renal injury or only a small renal contusion [96]. Similar findings of hematuria without obvious renal injury have been noted by others in series of pediatric patients with BAT [97]. It is important to note that gross hematuria is common in renal injuries, however, significant trauma can occur without the presence of gross or even microscopic hematuria, especially in cases involving complete disruption of the kidney from the ureter [12, 98].

As with spleen and liver injuries, nonoperative management is successful in the vast majority of cases of blunt renal trauma. Higher grade injuries, with disruption of the collecting system may require early intervention, either endoscopically, with placement of stents across the disruption(s) or with direct surgical repair [99]. Absolute indications for intervention include persistent hemodynamic instability due to bleeding and suspected ureteropelvic junction disruption with active urine leak [99].

## Diaphragmatic Injuries

Although relatively uncommon, diaphragmatic injuries resulting in herniation of abdominal contents into the thoracic cavity can occur with blunt abdominal forces in children. Because the energy required to create such an injury is significant, these cases are almost always associated with significant other injuries leading to higher overall injury severity and higher risk of ultimate mortality [100-102]. Reported mechanisms of injury include motor vehicle and all-terrain vehicle injuries, pedestrian-versus-truck, and run-over by truck injuries, suggesting major compressive forces [100, 102]. Risk of herniation appears to be more prevalent on the left, theorizing that the liver is somewhat protective on the right [101, 102], although one large series found both sides to be equally at risk [100]. Bilateral injuries can occur, although much more likely with penetrating mechanisms versus blunt forces.

Diagnosis can be made in over half of patients on chest radiographs, with evidence of intestinal loops in the thorax. However, in up to half of cases this may not be so obvious where significant blunt forces have occurred to result in other severe injuries. Chest x-ray may demonstrate features associated with diaphragmatic injury (indistinct or elevated hemidiaphragm, rib fractures, pneumothoraces, hemothoraces, pleural effusions), however CT scan with 3-dimensional reconstruction is recommended [101]. In unstable patients in whom imaging cannot be obtained, careful examination of the diaphragm should be done to rule out diaphragmatic injuries.

Surgical approach to this injury is predicated on need to assess and manage associated injuries. In most cases, careful repair through the abdomen with interrupted non-absorbable sutures can be done. A thoracic approach is often favored for right-sided injuries if laparotomy is not mandated. Associated major vascular injuries, especially with injuries on the right which may be associated with hepatic venous injuries, may require a thoracoabdominal approach. The choice of open versus minimally invasive approaches is dependent on the technical expertise available and need to address other injuries; both have been described in children [103, 104].

## Major Vascular Injuries

Being relatively protected in the mid-portion of the retroperitoneum, major vascular injuries with blunt forces, especially to the abdominal aorta, are extremely rare in children. One of the largest recent series by Hamner et al. reported 2.5% of children with blunt trauma reported in the US National Trauma Database having a major intraabdominal arterial injury, the vast majority of these as the result of motor vehicle collisions or pedestrian trauma [105]. Of these about one third involved the renal artery and less than one quarter involved mesenteric arteries and iliac arteries, each. Five percent were reported as aortic injuries; less than 0.1% of all cases of blunt abdominal injuries in children.

Undoubtedly, aortic injuries can cause significant concern to any physician faced with this injury in the pediatric population due to its rarity as well as high risk of associated mortality, often due to the multiple other associated injuries [105]. They are usually the result of acute compressive forces against the spine, with the vast majority of reported cases resulting from lap belt mechanisms, often in conjunction with a Chance fracture and abdominal wall and intraabdominal injuries as described earlier [16, 106]. Direct compression resulting from bicycle handlebars, all-terrain vehicle flips and non-accidental trauma have also been reported [16, 106]. Requiring a significant amount of force to occur, patients presenting to the ED with an abdominal aortic injury will almost always have some signs or symptoms. Any child presenting with a lap belt injury must be considered at risk, usually presenting with back and/or abdominal pain. More direct signs include relative ischemia to either or both lower extremities which may be overt with or without neurologic compromise or limited to reduced pulses.

If hemodynamically stable, CT scan with intravenous contrast may demonstrate aortic injuries. If hemodynamically unstable, and bleeding from sources other than the abdomen can be quickly ruled out, laparotomy is mandatory. Frank intraperitoneal bleeding from the aorta is unlikely to be encountered as such an injury would usually result in demise at the scene. Bleeding into the retroperitoneum with a contained hematoma may be seen at laparotomy, and if it is expanding, immediate intervention is required. A non-expanding retroperitoneal hematoma seen at laparotomy mandates further investigation to determine need for management.

Both direct and endovascular techniques have been described to repair abdominal aortic injuries in children; observation without intervention has also been reported [15, 107]. Joint decision making between pediatric surgery and vascular surgery to do what is in the best interest of the child [15], dependent upon other injuries is ideal in these complex and uncommon cases.

## Conclusion

Blunt trauma to children remains commonplace and when associated with significant energy or direct blows, significant intraabdominal injuries can occur. Accurate diagnosis and assessment of the injured child requires a systematic approach with a knowledge and heightened awareness of common injury patterns. Suspicion of specific injuries should guide workup; knowledge of expertise and resources will guide management. Unless associated with hollow organ or major vascular injuries, most children sustaining BAT can be managed without operative intervention. Careful monitoring by the astute physician with an understanding of the natural history of many of these injuries will direct care and ensure optimal outcomes.

## References

[1] World Health Organization. World report on child injury prevention. http://www.refworks.com/refworks2/?r=references|MainLayout::init. Updated 2008. Accessed June, 2015.

[2] Borisch B. An invisible epidemic: Preventing unintentional injuries among children and youth – A priority for national public health associations. . 2012;33:132.

[3] Public Health Agency of Caanda. Leading causes of death and hospitalization in canada. http://www.phac-aspc.gc.ca/publicat/lcd-pcd97/. Updated 2008. Accessed June, 2015.

[4] World Health Organization. 10 facts on youth and road safety. http://www.who.int/features/factfiles/youth_roadsafety/en/. Updated 2012. Accessed June, 2015.

[5] Hynick NH, Brennan M, Schmit P, Noseworthy S, Yanchar NL. Identification of blunt abdominal injuries in children. *J Trauma Acute Care Surg*. 2014;76(1):95-100.

[6] Lane WG, Dubowitz H, Langenberg P, Dischinger P. Epidemiology of abusive abdominal trauma hospitalizations in united states children. *Child Abuse Negl*. 2012;36(2):142-148.

[7] Santschi M, Lemoine C, Cyr C. The spectrum of seat belt syndrome among canadian children: Results of a two-year population surveillance study. *Paediatr Child Health*. 2008;13(4):279-283.

[8] Achildi O, Betz RR, Grewal H. Lapbelt injuries and the seatbelt syndrome in pediatric spinal cord injury. *J Spinal Cord Med*. 2007;30 Suppl 1:S21-4.

[9] Borgialli DA, Ellison AM, Ehrlich P, et al. Association between the seat belt sign and intra-abdominal injuries in children with blunt torso trauma in motor vehicle collisions. *Acad Emerg Med*. 2014;21(11):1240-1248.

[10] Shepherd M, Hamill J, Segedin E. Paediatric lap-belt injury: A 7 year experience. *Emerg Med Australas*. 2006;18(1):57-63.

[11] Griffet J, Bastiani-Griffet F, El-Hayek T, Dageville C, Pebeyre B. Management of seat-belt syndrome in children. gravity of 2-point seat-belt. *Eur J Pediatr Surg*. 2002;12(1):63-66.

[12] Santucci RA, Langenburg SE, Zachareas MJ. Traumatic hematuria in children can be evaluated as in adults. *J Urol*. 2004;171(2 Pt 1):822-825.

[13] Bruny JL, Bensard DD. Hollow viscous injury in the pediatric patient. *Semin Pediatr Surg*. 2004;13(2):112-118.

[14] Jones VS, Soundappan SV, Cohen RC, et al. Posttraumatic small bowel obstruction in children. *J Pediatr Surg*. 2007;42(8):1386-1388.

[15] Parrish DW, Barnhorst A, Trebska-McGowan K, Amendola M, Haynes JH. Nonoperative management of pediatric aortic injury with seat belt syndrome. *Ann Vasc Surg*. 2015.

[16] Choit RL, Tredwell SJ, Leblanc JG, Reilly CW, Mulpuri K. Abdominal aortic injuries associated with chance fractures in pediatric patients. *J Pediatr Surg*. 2006;41(6):1184-1190.
[17] Cherniawsky H, Bratu I, Rankin T, Sevcik WB. Serious impact of handlebar injuries. *Clin Pediatr (Phila)*. 2014;53(7):672-676.
[18] Dai LN, Chen CD, Lin XK, et al. Abdominal injuries involving bicycle handlebars in 219 children: Results of 8-year follow-up. *Eur J Trauma Emerg Surg*. 2014.
[19] Sutherland I, Ledder O, Crameri J, et al. Pancreatic trauma in children. *Pediatr Surg Int*. 2010;26(12):1201-1206.
[20] Nataraja RM, Palmer CS, Arul GS, Bevan C, Crameri J. The full spectrum of handlebar injuries in children: A decade of experience. *Injury*. 2014;45(4):684-689.
[21] Trokel M, Discala C, Terrin NC, Sege RD. Patient and injury characteristics in abusive abdominal injuries. *Pediatr Emerg Care*. 2006;22(10):700-704.
[22] Sowrey L, Lawson KA, Garcia-Filion P, et al. Duodenal injuries in the very young: Child abuse? *J Trauma Acute Care Surg*. 2013;74(1):136-41; discussion 141-2.
[23] Gaines BA, Shultz BS, Morrison K, Ford HR. Duodenal injuries in children: Beware of child abuse. *J Pediatr Surg*. 2004;39(4):600-602.
[24] Menaker J, Blumberg S, Wisner DH, et al. Use of the focused assessment with sonography for trauma (FAST) examination and its impact on abdominal computed tomography use in hemodynamically stable children with blunt torso trauma. *J Trauma Acute Care Surg*. 2014;77(3):427-432.
[25] Holmes JF, Mao A, Awasthi S, McGahan JP, Wisner DH, Kuppermann N. Validation of a prediction rule for the identification of children with intra-abdominal injuries after blunt torso trauma. *Ann Emerg Med*. 2009;54(4):528-533.
[26] Adelgais KM, Kuppermann N, Kooistra J, et al. Accuracy of the abdominal examination for identifying children with blunt intra-abdominal injuries. *J Pediatr*. 2014;165(6):1230-1235.e5.
[27] Acker SN, Stewart CL, Roosevelt GE, Partrick DA, Moore EE, Bensard DD. When is it safe to forgo abdominal CT in blunt-injured children? *Surgery*. 2015.
[28] Capraro AJ, Mooney D, Waltzman ML. The use of routine laboratory studies as screening tools in pediatric abdominal trauma. *Pediatr Emerg Care*. 2006;22(7):480-484.

[29] Sola JE, Cheung MC, Yang R, et al. Pediatric FAST and elevated liver transaminases: An effective screening tool in blunt abdominal trauma. *J Surg Res.* 2009;157(1):103-107.
[30] Holmes JF, Gladman A, Chang CH. Performance of abdominal ultrasonography in pediatric blunt trauma patients: A meta-analysis. *J Pediatr Surg.* 2007;42(9):1588-1594.
[31] Holmes JF, Sokolove PE, Brant WE, et al. Identification of children with intra-abdominal injuries after blunt trauma. *Ann Emerg Med.* 2002;39(5):500-509.
[32] Holmes JF, Lillis K, Monroe D, et al. Identifying children at very low risk of clinically important blunt abdominal injuries. *Ann Emerg Med.* 2013;62(2):107-116.e2.
[33] Pinto F, Miele V, Scaglione M, Pinto A. The use of contrast-enhanced ultrasound in blunt abdominal trauma: Advantages and limitations. *Acta Radiol.* 2014;55(7):776-784.
[34] Menichini G, Sessa B, Trinci M, Galluzzo M, Miele V. Accuracy of contrast-enhanced ultrasound (CEUS) in the identification and characterization of traumatic solid organ lesions in children: A retrospective comparison with baseline US and CE-MDCT. *Radiol Med.* 2015.
[35] Hom J. The risk of intra-abdominal injuries in pediatric patients with stable blunt abdominal trauma and negative abdominal computed tomography. *Acad Emerg Med.* 2010;17(5):469-475.
[36] Brenner D, Elliston C, Hall E, Berdon W. Estimated risks of radiation-induced fatal cancer from pediatric CT. *AJR Am J Roentgenol.* 2001;176(2):289-296.
[37] Miglioretti DL, Johnson E, Williams A, et al. The use of computed tomography in pediatrics and the associated radiation exposure and estimated cancer risk. *JAMA Pediatr.* 2013;167(8):700-707.
[38] Cohen MD. ALARA, image gently and CT-induced cancer. *Pediatr Radiol.* 2015;45(4):465-470.
[39] Callahan MJ. CT dose reduction in practice. *Pediatr Radiol.* 2011;41 Suppl 2:488-492.
[40] Khasawneh R, Ramakrishnaiah RH, Singh S, Hegde SV. CT findings in pediatric blunt intestinal injury. *Emerg Radiol.* 2013;20(6):545-552.
[41] Newman KD, Bowman LM, Eichelberger MR, et al. The lap belt complex: Intestinal and lumbar spine injury in children. *J Trauma.* 1990;30(9):1133-8; discussion 1138-40.

[42] Thompson SR, Holland AJ. Perforating small bowel injuries in children: Influence of time to operation on outcome. *Injury*. 2005;36(9):1029-1033.

[43] Ozturk H, Onen A, Otcu S, et al. Diagnostic delay increases morbidity in children with gastrointestinal perforation from blunt abdominal trauma. *Surg Today*. 2003;33(3):178-182.

[44] Streck CJ, Lobe TE, Pietsch JB, Lovvorn HN,3rd. Laparoscopic repair of traumatic bowel injury in children. *J Pediatr Surg*. 2006;41(11):1864-1869.

[45] Hamill J. Damage control surgery in children. *Injury*. 2004;35(7):708-712.

[46] Upadhyaya P. Conservative management of splenic trauma: History and current trends. *Pediatr Surg Int*. 2003;19(9-10):617-627.

[47] Upadhyaya P, Simpson JS. Splenic trauma in children. *Surg Gynecol Obstet*. 1968;126(4):781-790.

[48] Liu S, Bowman SM, Smith TC, Sharar SR. Trends in pediatric spleen management: Do hospital type and ownership still matter? *J Trauma Acute Care Surg*. 2015;78(5):935-942.

[49] Murphy EE, Murphy SG, Cipolle MD, Tinkoff GH. The pediatric trauma center and the inclusive trauma system: Impact on splenectomy rates. *J Trauma Acute Care Surg*. 2015;78(5):930-3; discussion 933-4.

[50] Polites SF, Zielinski MD, Zarroug AE, Wagie AE, Stylianos S, Habermann EB. Benchmarks for splenectomy in pediatric trauma: How are we doing? *J Pediatr Surg*. 2015;50(2):339-342.

[51] Stylianos S. Compliance with evidence-based guidelines in children with isolated spleen or liver injury: A prospective study. *J Pediatr Surg*. 2002;37(3):453-456.

[52] Bruce PJ, Helmer SD, Harrison PB, Sirico T, Haan JM. Nonsurgical management of blunt splenic injury: Is it cost effective? *Am J Surg*. 2011;202(6):810-5; discussion 815-6.

[53] Kristoffersen KW, Mooney DP. Long-term outcome of nonoperative pediatric splenic injury management. *J Pediatr Surg*. 2007;42(6):1038-41; discussion 1041-2.

[54] Thompson SR, Holland AJ. Evolution of non-operative management for blunt splenic trauma in children. *J Paediatr Child Health*. 2006;42(5):231-234.

[55] Aidonopoulos AP, Papavramidis ST, Goutzamanis GD, Filos GG, Deligiannidis NP, Vogiatzis IM. Splenorrhaphy for splenic damage in patients with multiple injuries. *Eur J Surg*. 1995;161(4):247-251.

[56] Steiner Z, Iuchtman M, Litmanovitch M, Breitgand A. Low morbidity profile of spleen mesh wrapping in children. *Eur J Pediatr Surg.* 2008;18(3):150-152.

[57] Lee J, Moriarty KP, Tashjian DB. Less is more: Management of pediatric splenic injury. *Arch Surg.* 2012;147(5):437-441.

[58] Li D, Yanchar N. Management of pediatric blunt splenic injuries in canada--practices and opinions. *J Pediatr Surg.* 2009;44(5):997-1004.

[59] Yang JC, Sharp SW, Ostlie DJ, Holcomb GW,3rd, St Peter SD. Natural history of nonoperative management for grade 4 and 5 liver and spleen injuries in children. *J Pediatr Surg.* 2008;43(12):2264-2267.

[60] Fremgen HE, Bratton SL, Metzger RR, Barnhart DC. Pediatric liver lacerations and intensive care: Evaluation of ICU triage strategies. *Pediatr Crit Care Med.* 2014;15(4):e183-91.

[61] Gross JL, Woll NL, Hanson CA, et al. Embolization for pediatric blunt splenic injury is an alternative to splenectomy when observation fails. *J Trauma Acute Care Surg.* 2013;75(3):421-425.

[62] Davies DA, Ein SH, Pearl R, et al. What is the significance of contrast "blush" in pediatric blunt splenic trauma? *J Pediatr Surg.* 2010;45(5):916-920.

[63] Cloutier DR, Baird TB, Gormley P, McCarten KM, Bussey JG, Luks FI. Pediatric splenic injuries with a contrast blush: Successful nonoperative management without angiography and embolization. *J Pediatr Surg.* 2004;39(6):969-971.

[64] Duron VP, Day KM, Steigman SA, Aidlen JT, Luks FI. Maintaining low transfusion and angioembolization rates in the age of nonoperative management of pediatric blunt splenic injury. *Am Surg.* 2014;80(11):1159-1163.

[65] Ong CC, Toh L, Lo RH, Yap TL, Narasimhan K. Primary hepatic artery embolization in pediatric blunt hepatic trauma. *J Pediatr Surg.* 2012;47(12):2316-2320.

[66] Vo NJ, Althoen M, Hippe DS, Prabhu SJ, Valji K, Padia SA. Pediatric abdominal and pelvic trauma: Safety and efficacy of arterial embolization. *J Vasc Interv Radiol.* 2014;25(2):215-220.

[67] Stylianos S. Evidence-based guidelines for resource utilization in children with isolated spleen or liver injury. the APSA trauma committee. *J Pediatr Surg.* 2000;35(2):164-7; discussion 167-9.

[68] St Peter SD, Aguayo P, Juang D, et al. Follow up of prospective validation of an abbreviated bedrest protocol in the management of blunt

spleen and liver injury in children. *J Pediatr Surg.* 2013;48(12):2437-2441.

[69] Davis DH, Localio AR, Stafford PW, Helfaer MA, Durbin DR. Trends in operative management of pediatric splenic injury in a regional trauma system. *Pediatrics.* 2005;115(1):89-94.

[70] Mooney DP, Rothstein DH, Forbes PW. Variation in the management of pediatric splenic injuries in the united states. *J Trauma.* 2006;61(2):330-3; discussion 333.

[71] McDonald LA, Yanchar NL. Management of pediatric splenic injuries in canada. *J Pediatr Surg.* 2012;47(3):473-476.

[72] Stylianos S, Egorova N, Guice KS, Arons RR, Oldham KT. Variation in treatment of pediatric spleen injury at trauma centers versus nontrauma centers: A call for dissemination of american pediatric surgical association benchmarks and guidelines. *J Am Coll Surg.* 2006;202(2):247-251.

[73] Sims CA, Wiebe DJ, Nance ML. Blunt solid organ injury: Do adult and pediatric surgeons treat children differently? *J Trauma.* 2008;65(3):698-703.

[74] Bowman SM, Sharar SR, Quan L. Impact of a statewide quality improvement initiative in improving the management of pediatric splenic injuries in washington state. *J Trauma.* 2008;64(6):1478-1483.

[75] Stylianos S. Outcomes from pediatric solid organ injury: Role of standardized care guidelines. *Curr Opin Pediatr.* 2005;17(3):402-406.

[76] Arkovitz MS, Johnson N, Garcia VF. Pancreatic trauma in children: Mechanisms of injury. *J Trauma.* 1997;42(1):49-53.

[77] Shilyansky J, Sena LM, Kreller M, et al. Nonoperative management of pancreatic injuries in children. *J Pediatr Surg.* 1998;33(2):343-349.

[78] Maeda K, Ono S, Baba K, Kawahara I. Management of blunt pancreatic trauma in children. *Pediatr Surg Int.* 2013;29(10):1019-1022.

[79] Mahajan A, Kadavigere R, Sripathi S, Rodrigues GS, Rao VR, Koteshwar P. Utility of serum pancreatic enzyme levels in diagnosing blunt trauma to the pancreas: A prospective study with systematic review. *Injury.* 2014;45(9):1384-1393.

[80] Cuenca AG, Islam S. Pediatric pancreatic trauma: Trending toward nonoperative management? *Am Surg.* 2012;78(11):1204-1210.

[81] Herman R, Guire KE, Burd RS, Mooney DP, Ehlrich PF. Utility of amylase and lipase as predictors of grade of injury or outcomes in pediatric patients with pancreatic trauma. *J Pediatr Surg.* 2011;46(5):923-926.

[82] Houben CH, Ade-Ajayi N, Patel S, et al. Traumatic pancreatic duct injury in children: Minimally invasive approach to management. *J Pediatr Surg*. 2007;42(4):629-635.

[83] Phelan HA, Velmahos GC, Jurkovich GJ, et al. An evaluation of multidetector computed tomography in detecting pancreatic injury: Results of a multicenter AAST study. *J Trauma*. 2009;66(3):641-6; discussion 646-7.

[84] Potoka DA, Gaines BA, Leppaniemi A, Peitzman AB. Management of blunt pancreatic trauma: What's new? *Eur J Trauma Emerg Surg*. 2015;41(3):239-250.

[85] Garvey EM, Haakinson DJ, McOmber M, Notrica DM. Role of ERCP in pediatric blunt abdominal trauma: A case series at a level one pediatric trauma center. *J Pediatr Surg*. 2015;50(2):335-338.

[86] Stringer MD. Pancreatic trauma in children. *Br J Surg*. 2005;92(4):467-470.

[87] Iqbal CW, St Peter SD, Tsao K, et al. Operative vs nonoperative management for blunt pancreatic transection in children: Multi-institutional outcomes. *J Am Coll Surg*. 2014;218(2):157-162.

[88] Beres AL, Wales PW, Christison-Lagay ER, McClure ME, Fallat ME, Brindle ME. Non-operative management of high-grade pancreatic trauma: Is it worth the wait? *J Pediatr Surg*. 2013;48(5):1060-1064.

[89] Sheikh F, Fallon S, Bisset G, et al. Image-guided prediction of pseudocyst formation in pediatric pancreatic trauma. *J Surg Res*. 2015;193(2):513-518.

[90] Abbo O, Lemandat A, Reina N, et al. Conservative management of blunt pancreatic trauma in children: A single center experience. *Eur J Pediatr Surg*. 2013;23(6):470-473.

[91] Cigdem MK, Senturk S, Onen A, Siga M, Akay H, Otcu S. Nonoperative management of pancreatic injuries in pediatric patients. *Surg Today*. 2011;41(5):655-659.

[92] Iqbal CW, Levy SM, Tsao K, et al. Laparoscopic versus open distal pancreatectomy in the management of traumatic pancreatic disruption. *J Laparoendosc Adv Surg Tech A*. 2012;22(6):595-598.

[93] Haugaard MV, Wettergren A, Hillingso JG, Gluud C, Penninga L. Non-operative versus operative treatment for blunt pancreatic trauma in children. *Cochrane Database Syst Rev*. 2014;2:CD009746.

[94] Brown SL, Elder JS, Spirnak JP. Are pediatric patients more susceptible to major renal injury from blunt trauma? A comparative study. *Journal of Urology*. 1998;160:138.

[95] Tojuola BD, Gu X, Littlejohn NR, Sharpe JP, Williams MA, Giel DW. Does the mechanism of injury in pediatric blunt trauma patients correlate with the severity of genitourinary organ injury? *Can J Urol.* 2014;21(6):7570-7573.
[96] Brown SL, Haas C, Dinchman KH, Elder JS, Spirnak JP. Radiologic evaluation of pediatric blunt renal trauma in patients with microscopic hematuria. *World J Surg.* 2001;25(12):1557-1560.
[97] Thorp AW, Young TP, Brown L. Test characteristics of urinalysis to predict urologic injury in children. *West J Emerg Med.* 2011;12(2):168-172.
[98] Perez-Brayfield MR, Gatti JM, Smith EA, et al. Blunt traumatic hematuria in children. is a simplified algorithm justified? *J Urol.* 2002;167(6):2543-6; discussion 2546-7.
[99] Reese JN, Fox JA, Cannon GM, Ost MC. Timing and predictors for urinary drainage in children with expectantly managed grade IV renal trauma. *J Urol.* 2014;192(2):512-7.
[100] Ramos CT, Koplewitz BZ, Babyn PS, Manson PS, Ein SH. What have we learned about traumatic diaphragmatic hernias in children? *J Pediatr Surg.* 2000;35(4):601-604.
[101] Okur MH, Uygun I, Arslan MS, et al. Traumatic diaphragmatic rupture in children. *J Pediatr Surg.* 2014;49(3):420-423.
[102] Al-Salem AH. Traumatic diaphragmatic hernia in children. *Pediatr Surg Int.* 2012;28(7):687-691.
[103] Gaines BA, Rutkoski JD. The role of laparoscopy in pediatric trauma. *Semin Pediatr Surg.* 2010;19(4):300-303.
[104] Parelkar SV, Oak SN, Patel JL, et al. Traumatic diaphragmatic hernia: Management by video assisted thoracoscopic repair. *J Indian Assoc Pediatr Surg.* 2012;17(4):180-183.
[105] Hamner CE, Groner JI, Caniano DA, Hayes JR, Kenney BD. Blunt intraabdominal arterial injury in pediatric trauma patients: Injury distribution and markers of outcome. *J Pediatr Surg.* 2008;43(5):916-923.
[106] McCarthy MC, Price SW, Rundell WK, et al. Pediatric blunt abdominal aortic injuries: Case report and review of the literature. *J Trauma.* 2007;63(6):1383-1387.
[107] Papazoglou KO, Karkos CD, Kalogirou TE, Giagtzidis IT. Endovascular management of lap belt-related abdominal aortic injury in a 9-year-old child. *Ann Vasc Surg.* 2015;29(2):365.e11-365.e15.

In: Abdominal Trauma ...
Editor: Louise Santiago

ISBN: 978-1-63483-482-7


*Chapter 2*

# Open Abdomen Management for Abdominal Trauma: Indications and Surgical Modalities

***Stefano Rausei*, Vincenzo Pappalardo, Francesco Amico, Francesco Frattini, Luigi Boni, Francesca Rovera and Gianlorenzo Dionigi***
Department of Surgery, University of Insubria, Varese, Italy

## Abstract

Open abdomen (OA) is a term currently used to refer to leaving abdominal incision open after surgical procedure. Indications for OA management are heterogeneous and consensus has not been reached to date. However, in trauma setting damage control surgery and abdominal compartment syndrome are the most common indications for such treatment. OA is usually managed with temporary abdominal closure (TAC) techniques. TAC is an attempt to control fluid losses, minimize the loss of domain, and to reduce fascial retraction. These techniques are also used as a bridge treatment to facilitate patient management until definitive closure is obtained. OA management is a result of a conjunct effort of surgeons and anesthesiologists. Such collaboration could also

* Corresponding author: Stefano Rausei, Department of Surgery, University of Insubria, Varese, Italy, Mail address: via F. Guicciardini 9, 21100 Varese, Email: stefano.rausei@ospedale.varese.it, Fax: +39.332.260260, Phone: +39.349.8535.931.

increase any possibility to produce high quality evidence in this field: in fact, an agreement about the right timing and method for abdominal closure is still to be obtained. A literature review will be presented to try to clarify crucial aspects of this topic.

## INTRODUCTION

In this chapter we will discuss open abdomen (OA), its meaning, evolution, indications and management in trauma patients. We will analyze different treatment aspects including methods no longer in use and will focus on new methods that showed encouraging results.

## HISTORICAL FOREWORD

OA is a treatment for which the surgeon, by necessity or in the context of a well-planned strategy, does not proceed with the conventional synthesis of the abdominal fascia after surgical procedure. Hence, this term is currently used to refer to an abdominal wall defect with exposure of abdominal viscera. In the context of English literature, among the first authors reporting OA experiences, Ogilvie (during the Second World War) described a pioneering OA management.

"*A dodge that has twice helped me in a difficulty is the use of light canvas or stout cotton cloth sterilized in Vaseline. A double sheet of this is cut rather smaller than the defect in the muscles and sutured into place with interrupted catgut sutures [...]. This device is obviously temporary, but it prevents retraction of the edges of the gap, it keeps the intestinal contents from protruding during the early days when they are so difficult to retain, and it allows the abdominal wall to be used as a whole in respiration*" [1].

In the early twentieth century Pringle described some forerunner damage control techniques in patients with severe hepatic trauma [2]. In 1969 Alexander J. Walt discussed his work to the Royal College of England arguing that there was no place in modern surgery for gauze packing of the liver as sepsis and recurrent bleeding were inevitable sequelae [3]. Nevertheless he was aware of the critically reduced reserves in surgical patients suffering hypotension, severe shock, acidosis, multiple injuries, thus further contributing to a cultural discussion in the scientific community. Several years later (1993), this probably brought Rotondo to define the landmark of damage control surgery (DCS) [4]. Initially, as often it happens, OA was an intuition dictated by necessity more then a well-weighted choice. Since then this method has undergone many changes and improvements and has now become indispensable for trauma surgeons.

## INDICATIONS

Each abdominal surgical procedure should conclude with muscular fascia closure, but when it is not possible (or not preferable) the surgeon is enforced to leave the abdomen open. Hence, the strategy of OA may be planned even before or during the operation. OA in trauma patients has several indications; most of them are related to DCS or Abdominal Compartment Syndrome (ACS) patterns.

### Damage Control Surgery

The terms DCS for trauma patients are defined as the rapid initial control of bleeding and contamination, temporary abdominal closure (TAC), resuscitation to normal physiology and subsequent re-explorations with definitive reconstruction procedures. The goal of DCS is to restore normal physiology before normal anatomy to prevent the "lethal triad" (coagulopathy, hypothermia and metabolic acidosis) [5]. In fact, a careful assessment (and follow-up) of the injuries and a safe control of bleeding often implies that abdomen must be left open. Usually, OA in trauma is indicated in the presence of packing for bleeding injuries or vascular/gastrointestinal injuries that need a second look. Sometimes, after trauma also the loss of abdominal wall associated with extensive contamination makes OA approach obligatory.

### Lethal Triad

This triad (hypothermia, acidosis and coagulopathy) in trauma is believed to be secondary to tissue hypoxia in states of hypovolaemia and subsequent inadequate tissue perfusion. This is a detrimental prognostic factor for traumatized patients [6, 7], but the implementation of DCS principles, during resuscitation and surgery, has enabled better outcomes.

Post-traumatic *hypothermia* is generally considered to be present in patients with a body core temperature below 35°C [8-10] and severe hypothermia is any temperature below 32°C. Hypothermia after injury is induced by either environmental exposure [11], infusion of cold fluids, or as a side-effect of anaesthetic drugs affecting thermoregulation [10, 12]. Mild heat loss is usually well tolerated, with compensatory pathophysiological changes to maintain temperature homeostasis [12]. Below 32°C, cardiac conduction disturbances become apparent; atrial fibrillation is seen in about half of all patients with a core temperature below 30°C. Serious abnormal cardiac rhythms start to occur below about 28°C [10, 12]. At core temperatures lower than 28°C, the respiratory rate dramatically decreases and myocardial contractility is depressed [13-16]. Hypothermia decreases the enzymatic activity of clotting factors and impairs platelet function. In addition, hypothermia inhibits fibrinogen synthesis [17, 18]. Anaerobic metabolism results in reduced adenosine 5-triphosphate (ATP) synthesis, leading to decreased hydrolysis of ATP to adenosine 5-diphosphate and decreased heat production [17]. Some authors argue that, within the most common temperature range seen in trauma patients (33–36°C), isolated hypothermia probably has only a minimal clinical impact on hemostasis [19]. Several studies have shown an independent relationship between death and hypothermia after trauma [20-27].

*Acidosis* is usually considered as an arterial pH below 7·36. The most clear indicator of metabolic acidosis in trauma is the increased serum concentration of lactate, produced as result of an increased anaerobic metabolism [28-30]. The role of metabolic acidosis in the lethal triad is complex. It is recognized as a marker of inadequate resuscitation and impending organ failure, but its direct relation to hypothermia and coagulopathy is not entirely clear, except that all three are believed mutually to perpetuate the state of shock preceding death in trauma. Even though acidosis is known to induce coagulopathy, an in vitro study on whole blood showed that, without the presence of hypothermia, the effect of acidosis was insignificant [31]. Acidosis decreases cardiac contractility, attenuates adrenergic receptor responsiveness to inotropic agents, impairs renal perfusion, and coagulation [32]. The propagation phase of thrombin generation is inhibited, the depletion of the platelet count occurs, and the activity of some coagulation factors (especially Xa/Va complex) is reduced. These manifest as prolonged clotting times and increased bleeding times [18, 33]. In addition, pH neutralization does not completely correct coagulation, implying some unknown effect of acidosis [33-35]. These factors provide strong evidence for acidosis as a major contributor to coagulopathy. Prognostically, acidosis during the first 24 h correlates significantly with post-injury organ failure and death [36], since it is associated also with lower cardiac performance [37]. Base excess has been reported to be the best detector of occult hypoperfusion (defined as hypoperfusion in the presence of normal vital signs) [38].

An understanding of *coagulopathy* in injured patients has evolved with time [39, 40]. By definition, if hemostasis is the control of bleeding without pathological thrombotic events [41], coagulopathy can be defined as any flaw in the coagulation system, leading to either increased bleeding time. The simple synergy of hypothermia and acidosis in a trauma setting leading to coagulopathy has been challenged [19, 39, 42, 43]. Rather than a secondary effect of dilution and consumption as was believed in the past, trauma-induced coagulopathy is currently considered to be a combination of primary (endogenous response) and secondary (caused by dilution and consumption) events [19, 43]. Acute traumatic coagulopathy is an impairment of hemostasis that occurs early after injury and develops endogenously in response to a combination of tissue damage and shock [42, 44]. It is associated with a fourfold higher mortality rate, increased transfusion requirement and an increased occurrence of organ failure [45-47]. Trauma-induced coagulopathy can lead to both diffuse bleeding and the formation of clots, resulting in microthrombosis. The condition resembles to disseminated intravascular coagulopathy, but with different initiators and underlying mechanisms [19]. Injuries induce perturbations in the coagulation system in many ways [48]. The protein C pathway seems to be an important contributor to trauma-induced coagulopathy when an injury is associated with hypoperfusion [44, 49]. Hypoperfusion induces expression of thrombomodulin on the endothelial cell wall. Following the thrombin burst, thrombin combines with thrombomodulin and the endothelial protein C receptor. This complex activates protein C, that probably plays an essential role by the inhibition of some coagulation factors for a definitive hypocoagulable and hyperfibrinolytic state [50-51]. The role of platelets in trauma is also not yet resolved. A major bleeding episode can be the result of an insufficient platelet levels. Thrombocytopenia at admission after trauma has been linked to increased mortality, and the highest survival rates are seen in patients receiving the highest platelet to erythrocyte ratio of transfusion [52]. Function is probably more important than the absolute platelet count. Platelet function is to some extent reflected by viscoelastic hemostatic assays and rotational thromboelastometry [53-54]. Platelets are probably the most important factors involved in early coagulation steps. Despite this, the role of platelets in trauma-induced coagulopathy is poorly investigated and management guidelines are not so clear [45, 55]. Actually, the trend in massive transfusion protocols worldwide has been towards the early addition of platelets in a ratio 1:1:1 for packed red blood cells, fresh frozen plasma, thrombocytes [56-58]. Additionally, primary fibrinolysis appears to be fundamental in trauma-induced coagulopathy and occurs early (less than 1 h) after trauma [18, 34, 59]. Fibrinolysis is associated with massive transfusion requirements, coagulopathy and hemorrhage-related death [60]. Trauma alters fibrinogen metabolism in a variety of ways [18]. Ongoing hemorrhage may cause accelerated fibrinogen breakdown. Loss of blood and decreases in core body temperature inhibit fibrinogen synthesis, and acidosis causes accelerated fibrinogen breakdown. In this regard, the test with thromboelastography seems crucial in identifying coagulation abnormalities at an early stage. A near linear relationship has been shown to exist between the degree of coagulopathy and increasing injuries scores [47]. This association is even stronger when adding hypothermia, acidosis and hypotension to severity of injury [61].

## Abdominal Compartment Syndrome

ACS is a pattern of altered cardiovascular haemodynamics, respiratory mechanics and renal function due to a sustained increase in intra-abdominal pressure (IAP; normal IAP is approximately 5–7 mm Hg in critically ill adults and urinary bladder pressure is the most used reference parameter). The terms ACS were proposed by Kron et al. in 1984 [62], but ACS was first suggested as an entity by Baggot in 1951 [63]. In ACS there is a compromission of renal, cardiac and respiratory functions (and lethal triad can occur), despite adequate fluid resuscitation and ventilation. Harman et al. [64] demonstrated that in an animal model the increase of IAP up to 20 mmHg involves a reduction of glomerular filtration rate and urine output. In fact, an IAP of 15-20 mmHg causes oliguria and an increase to 40 mmHg leads to anuria [64-66]. Compression of renal veins and kidneys seems to be the most likely cause of renal failure when ACS occurs [67, 68]. An increased IAP causes a decreased cardiac output and stroke volume as well as increased systemic vascular resistance (due to a low cardiac preload) [64, 66, 69] ACS also increases peak airway pressure and thoracic pleural pressure, thereby compromising ventilation in addition to decreasing cardiac output [70, 71]. Patients with ACS (defined as intra-abdominal pressure >20 mm Hg with organ dysfunction) often requires a decompressive laparotomy and in severe cases intra-abdominal hypertension persists after laparotomy; in fact, IAP should be monitored even during the OA. Although traditional threshold values for abdominal pressure and its relationship to intra-abdominal hypertension and ACS have been published, the diagnosis remains largely clinical: intra-abdominal hypertension without clinical signs cannot be considered ACS. Generally, intra-abdominal hypertension is defined by a sustained or repeated pathologic elevation of IAP≥12 mm Hg and an IAP >25 mmHg often is associated with ACS (Table 1).

**Table 1. Classification of intra-abdominal hypertension**

| | |
|---|---|
| Grade I | 12–15 mm Hg |
| Grade II | 16–20 mm Hg |
| Grade III | 21–25 mm Hg |
| Grade IV | >25 mmHg |

**Table 2. Predictive factors for ACS**

| |
|---|
| pH <7.2 |
| Core temperature <34°C |
| Estimated blood loss >4L |
| Systolic blood pressure <70 mmHg |
| Lactate levels (LA) > 5 mmol/L |
| Base deficit (BD) > -6 in patients > 55 years of age or > -15 in patients < 55 years of age |
| Prothrombin time > 1.6 |

A considerable amount of traumatized patients are at risk of developing ACS [72, 73] as result of visceral or retroperitoneal swelling, recurrent bleeding and intra-peritoneal packing [74, 75]. Decompressive laparotomy is indicated when medical treatment fails to resolve ACS and there are increasing signs of organ failure or impending lethal triad. This scenario occurs in critical patients, which already present some predictive factors like alteration of pH, blood pressure, lactate levels (Table 2) [73]. For this reason, OA is a treatment of choice for clear ACS, but also for prevention of ACS in trauma patients with specific risk factors. Therefore, preventive OA could be indicated for these situations: 1) DCS and planned reoperation within a day or two; 2) retroperitoneal or visceral swelling with elevated IAP; 3) difficult abdominal high-tension closure. Lastly, OA technique should be considered if the patient is receiving massive transfusion (≥10 units packed RBCs). It should be remembered that some experts indicate OA as treatment also for refractory intracranial hypertension associated with multi-compartment syndrome.

## How to Remember OA Indications?

The following table (Table 3) is an aid to clarify all the different indications for OA management in trauma patients [72-75], categorized according to the "common sense" by Moshe Schein [76].

**Table 3. Indications for OA management in trauma patients categorized according to the "common sense" by Schein [76]**

| |
|---|
| **When the abdomen cannot be closed** |
| Major abdominal tissue loss |
| Poor fascia conditions |
| Extreme visceral or retroperitoneal swelling |
| Elevated bladder pressure (IAP) after surgery during the closure of the fascia |
| **When the abdomen should not be close** |
| Planned reoperation within a day or two |
| Failure of medical treatment of ACS |
| Lesions causing hemorrhages from any organ in the peritoneal cavity possibly needing packing |
| Lesions involving the lumen of the gastrointestinal tract causing peritoneal contamination |
| Lesions to the small bowel mesentery conditioning increased ischemic risk for the pertaining small bowel tract |
| Pancreatic injury grade IV-V and injury of biliary tree |
| Patients requiring large volume resuscitation (>15 L or >10 Units of PRBCs) |

# Classification

The context of OA management always involves very critical patients and managing any patient with an OA is per se a great challenge, even in the hands of an experienced surgeon. After this premise, a classification for OA could be useful to the surgeon to better understand any possible scenario and then implement the best surgical treatment solution, but the focus must remain the patient, not the abdomen alone.

The simple and clear classification reported by Björck et al. [77] (Table 4) categorized the OA within this complex patient population according to some surgical criteria (i.e., adhesions, fixity, fistula). It could be useful to prevent further deterioration of the surgical field during treatment and appropriately maintain it at the lowest classification's grade to facilitate a primary delayed fascial closure as quickly as possible, but only when clinically appropriate.

**Table 4. Bjork classification of open abdomen [76]**

| | |
|---|---|
| **1a** | Clean OA without adherence between bowel and abdominal wall or fixity (lateralization of abdominal wall) |
| **1b** | Contaminated OA without adherence or fixity |
| **2a** | Clean OA developing adherence or fixity |
| **2b** | Contaminated OA developing adherence or fixity |
| **3** | OA complicated by fistula |
| **4** | Frozen abdomen |

## TEMPORARY ABDOMINAL CLOSURE TECHNIQUES

Delayed abdominal closure has revolutionized the care of the critically ill trauma and surgical patients who cannot tolerate primary abdominal closure. OA requires to be managed with TAC techniques: they refer to the decision to leave the abdomen open and the subsequent need to cover the abdominal defect.

Several techniques are available for this aim (Table 5) [78-85]. After a TAC period, the abdominal fascia must be closed as soon as possible. In fact, the first goal should remain delayed primary fascial closure. Any surgeon should know that the healing process of the abdominal wound allows only a limited window of opportunity for early closure (generally, within 10 days). The window starts when the visceral edema subsides and stops when the peritoneal space between the viscera and the abdominal wall becomes obliterated from adhesions. Meanwhile, lateral retraction of wound edges results in a progressively larger gap in the fascia.

**Table 5. Overview and characteristics of TAC techniques (modified by Boele van Hensbroek P et al. [77])**

| Technique | Description | Mechanism |
|---|---|---|
| Vacuum-assisted closure | A perforated plastic sheet covers the viscera and a sponge is placed between the facial edges. The wound is covered by an airtight seal, which is pierced by a suction drain that is connected to a suction pump and fluid collection system. | The (active and adjustable) negative pressure supplied by the pump keeps constant tension on the fascial edges while it collects excess abdominal fluid and helps to resolve edema. |
| Vacuum pack | A perforated plastic sheet covers the viscera, damp surgical towels are placed in the wound, and a surgical drain is placed on the towels. An airtight seal covers the wound and negative pressure is applied through the drain. | The negative pressure keeps constant tension on the fascial edges and excess fluid is collected. |
| Artificial burr (Wittmann patch) | Two opposite Velcro sheets (hooks and loops, one on each side) are sutured to the fascial edges. The Velcro sheets connect in the middle. | This technique allows for easy access and stepwise re-approximation of the fascial edges. |
| Dynamic retention sutures | The viscera are covered with a sheet. Horizontal sutures are placed through a large-diameter catheter and through entire abdominal wall on both sides. | The sutures keep tension on the fascia and may be tightened to allow staged re-approximation of the fascial edges. May be combined with a vacuum system. |
| Plastic silo (Bogota´ bag) | A sterile X-ray film cassette bag or sterile 3-L urology irrigation bag is sutured between the fascial edges or the skin and opened in the middle. | An easy technique that allows for easy access. The bag may be reduced in size to approximate the fascial edges. |
| Mesh | An absorbable or non-absorbable mesh or sheet is sutured between the fascial edges. | The mesh may be reduced in size to allow for re-approximation. Non-absorbable meshes may be removed or left in place at the end of the open abdominal period. |
| Loose packing | The fascial defect is covered by standard wound dressing only. | This technique is simple but does not prevent fascial retraction. |
| Zipper | A mesh or sheet with a sterilized zipper is sutured between the fascial edges. | This technique is comparable to the mesh/sheet and allows for easy access. |

| Technique | Description | Mechanism |
|---|---|---|
| Skin approximation | The skin is closed over the fascial defect with towel clips or a running suture. | Skin provides a "natural cover" for the viscera, but the towel clips obstruct radiological imaging and do not prevent fascial retraction. |

Therefore, the techniques of TAC may influence survival, number and severity of complications, timing for definitive fascial closure as well as future quality of life of patients. The ideal TAC technique should prevent ACS, should be quickly applied, easily changed, should contain and protect the abdominal viscera thus preventing loss of domain, decrease bowel edema, limit contamination, allow egress of peritoneal fluid (and its estimation) and not result in adhesions. It also should be cost-effective, minimizing both number of dressing changes and operative room access, resulting in a high rate of early closure with a low rate of complications, particularly enteroatmospheric fistula. At the same time an ideal TAC system should allow a correct management of oostomies on the abdominal wall. In fact, both ileostomy and colostomy could interfere with the proper placement of the dressing and lead to leakage of bowel contents onto the open wound. Delayed stoma maturation is advisable when possible as it makes it easier to manage the temporary closed abdomen.

Conventionally, available options for TAC can be categorized in skin approximation techniques (towel clip closure, the Bogota's bag, the silo technique) [86, 87]; fascial closure techniques, using an interposed material sutured to the abdominal fascia (e.g., the Wittmann Patch; absorbable or non-absorbable meshes) [88]; negative pressure wound therapy (NPWT) (Barker's vacuum pack, VAC Abdominal Dressing System, ABThera, Renasys) (Table 5) [89-94]. Skin techniques have been abandoned because of high complication rates. Both the Bogota's bag and the silo technique are prone to evisceration, do not prevent wall retraction and do not allow effective egress of peritoneal fluid with a poor nursing management. Moreover, the artificial material limits the expansion of the abdominal content to a fixed volume, with subsequent risk of ACS development and fistula formation [73]. Fascial closure techniques with using patch techniques consist in the interposition by suture of a prosthetic material between the edges of the abdominal fascia. Wittman patch and polytetrafluoroethylene (PTFE) patch are two main options used to achieve abdominal closure and allow easy re-entry into the abdomen. The Wittman patch sheet is sutured to the abdominal fascia laterally and closed at the midline with velcro like adjustable suture. Even if these methods limit the loss of domain due to fascial edge retraction, they do not prevent adhesions between viscera and the abdominal wall, while increasing the risk of fascial trauma. Moreover, these techniques do not allow the evacuation of peritoneal fluid. Additionally, interposed absorbable meshes are used to approximate and thus form a bed of granulation tissue for future skin grafting. Their most significant drawbacks are the low rate of primary closure and the high rate of fistula formation with non-absorbable graft [95, 96].

## Negative Pressure Wound Therapy

Brock introduced the vacuum pack technique in 1995 [97]. This technique used a three-layer device: 1) a fenestrated polyvinyl sheet draped over the exposed viscera and tucked under the fascial edges; 2) a surgical towel placed under the fascia followed by two silicone drains on top of the towel; 3) an adhesive, iodophorimpregnated polyester drape placed over the skin laterally to the anterior axillary lines to seal the wound. The drains are then connected to wall suction, with a 100–150 mmHg continuous negative pressure. Authors reported the main advantage of the prevention of injury to the abdominal wall by not suturing it, but preserving it for later closure [98, 99]. It also appeared safe, inexpensive, and effective for control of fluid loss. A disadvantage of the technique was that the prevention of loss of abdominal domain seems limited and its primary fascial closure rate was not satisfactory (about 50%) [100]. A relevant modification of the vacuum pack was described by Garner et al. and Miller et al. the vacuum-assisted fascial closure or the vacuum-assisted wound closure [101, 102]. This system resembles to the later developed devices, commercially available today. In these first studies, they used a polyurethane sponge over a non-adhesive polyethylene sheet and used a special pump as the vacuum source instead of wall suction. They also attempted partial suturing of the abdominal wall, placing sutures at the proximal and distal edges after each procedure, and subsequently used smaller pieces of foam. In 2004, the same group presented the results of a prospective study of 53 trauma patients treated with vacuum-assisted fascial closure in a standardized treatment algorithm. They achieved an 88% closure rate [103]. For patients with an OA, negative pressure systems specifically designed for use as a TAC method with a visceral protective layer (ABThera Active Abdominal Therapy, KCI, Acelity company, and RENASYS™ AB Abdominal Dressing Kit, Smith&Nephew) have also been developed. A commercialised system is now available that combines NPWT with intermittent instillation of a topical wound solution with a dwell time (NPWTi-d, VAC VeraFlo Therapy, KCI, Acelity company) for wounds that would benefit from controlled automated wound cleaning.The highest rates of primary fascial closure seem to be reached with a combination of NPWT and dynamic closure system (e.g., mediated retention sutures) [104, 105].

The optimal therapeutic level of negative pressure that seems to maximize tissue growth is about 100-125 mmHg. If active bleeding due to coagulopathy is suspected, the pressure level has to be lower, about 75 mmHg [96].

## Effects of NPWT

The events underlying the improvement in wound healing observed after use of NPWT can be classified as primary mechanisms and secondary effects. Four primary mechanisms of action have been proposed: 1) wound shrinkage or macrodeformation; 2) microdeformation at the foam-wound surface interface; 3) fluid removal; and 4) stabilization of the wound environment [106]. Secondary effects include angiogenesis, neurogenesis, granulation tissue formation, cellular proliferation, differentiation and migration [107].

## Advantages of NWPT in OA Management

NPWT has several potential advantages in OA setting and seems to allow to achieve all the goals suggested for an ideal TAC system.

***1) Protection of Exposed Organs, Reduction of Adhesions between the Bowel and Abdominal Wall and Decrease of Risk of Fistula***

A key treatment goal for the use of NPWT in early phases of OA is to prevent deterioration of the surgical field in terms of adhesions and fixity. With this purpose, all commercial NPWT devices contain a dedicated interface layer as part of the kit. It use a large, fenestrated non-adherent interface layer reducing adhesions between the exposed bowel and the abdominal wall, thus retaining the option of fascial closure. Application of this interface layer can reduce the risk of enteroatmospheric fistula [108], as prevention of adhesions leads to lower risk of bowel damage. Technically, the interface layer should be placed as widely as possible inside the abdomen: laterally into the paracolic gutters, cranially onto the diaphragm after taking down the falciform ligament and caudally into the pelvic cavity.

### *2) Fluids Drainage, Estimation and Identification of Their Quality, Prevention of ACS, Reduction of Analgesia, Contamination, Dressing Changes, Skin's Maceration, Heat Loss, Evaporative Fluid Loss and Edema*

A major advantage of NPWT over the other TAC techniques is its ability to actively drain fluids and to maintain low IAP preventing ACS, as results of the application of negative pressure. Certainly, it reduces the contamination of the abdominal cavity. In fact, from OA wounds treated with NPWT large volumes of fluids (about 800ml) can be evacuated [109]. Again, this better fluid handling may reduce the frequency of the operative room access with implications on sedation and analgesia and can prevent complications secondary to lying in wet beds. All evacuated fluids are directed into a waste canister preventing contamination of the ward and personal and maceration of the surrounding skin. Measurement of the fluid in the canister is easily carried out and may contribute to more rapid fluid replacement and nutritional support. Also, quick identification of the fluid quality (such as blood or bilioenteric material) can be easily observed through the transparent canister. Furthermore, in an animal model of OA, NPWT was shown to significantly reduce intestinal edema compared with passive drainage [110]. Although this has not been well confirmed clinically in the OA, maintaining the abdomen in a moist environment as a result of the NPWT top layer adhesive film also prevents uncontrolled evaporative fluid loss and reduces heat loss.

### *3) Preparation to Definitive Fascial Closure, Fast and Safe Healing of Wound*

In experienced hands NPWT should be used as a first line therapy in early phases of OA management for a more likely delayed primary closure. Hence, in wounds with a high probability of definitive fascial closure (such as some ACS and trauma-derived OA cases without substance loss), use of NPWT can be recommended over the other available methods of TAC. Firstly, unlike Wittmann patch and other zipper or mesh based techniques, NPWT is a suture-less technology and its application does not damage the fascial tissue. Secondly, unlike the Bogota bag approach, NPWT helps to prevent loss of abdominal domain in addition to providing active fluid drainage. Finally, the fewer explorative procedures reduce surgical trauma on the native fascia and improve fascial closure rates. In a study, patients closed at the first re-laparotomy were more likely to have been managed with NPWT and NPWT was an independent predictor for this early closure [111]. Another study reported that 43% of trauma patients with OA required only a single application of NPWT before fascial closure [112].

Once closure of the fascia and skin have been achieved, it is possible to use NPWT to support healing of the closed laparotomy incision and prevent complications. A significant reduction in wound complications (including dehiscence) was observed compared with standard gauze dressings in some comparative studies [113]. NPWT has also been used to support healing of high risk abdominal incisions in procedures where the abdomen is closed at the index operation [114, 115]. The application of NPWT is also believed to aid patient mobility, important in reducing duration of hospitalization and improving long-term outcomes [105]. The use of NPWT on closed incisions has been demonstrated to good effect in other clinical indications. Data from some studies can be extrapolated to provide further support to its likely efficacy in healing of 'at risk' laparotomy incisions [116-120].

***4) Reduction of Fistula Rate, Management of Fistula***

Fistulas in OA field are not so rare. They have some well-known risk factors (Table 6). Potential intestinal fistula mechanisms are anastomotic or stump leakage, traumatized or ischemic bowel, pressure ulceration or rupture in case of distal obstruction. A fistula opening directly from the bowel into an OA field is known as an entero-atmospheric fistula. The key components of management of the patient with an entero-atmospheric fistula are nutritional support, output and sepsis control, and local wound care [121-126]. More than 50% of patient with intestinal fistulas will need surgery for the control of sepsis and subsequent surgical repair for failure to close spontaneously [127, 128]. Nutritional support, either enteral or parenteral, is considered a critical measure to prevent malnutrition in an already critically debilitated patient [129].

**Table 6. Risk factors for fistula formation in OA**

| |
|---|
| Presence of bowel injury and repairs or anastomosis |
| Colon resection during DCS |
| Large fluid resuscitation volume (>10L/48hrs) |
| Presence of intra-abdominal sepsis/abscess |
| Number of re-explorations |
| Delayed abdominal closure >8 days |
| Polypropylene mesh directly over the bowel |

Nutritional support has to be through enteral feeding whenever possible. It should be started as soon as possible in order to prevent malnutrition. The only contraindication to enteral nutrition is an usable bowel shorter than 75 cm [124]. A standard polymeric formula supplying a daily intake of 20-30 Kcal/Kg of nonprotein calories with 1.5-2.5 g/kg of proteins is indicated to obtain a positive nitrogen balance. A high-output fistula is likely to require 1.5-2 times the usual calories because of ongoing losses [125]. The definitive treatment of fistulas has to be performed when the patient has fully recovered and in good nutritional status, usually after 6-12 months. Surgical repair, by suturing although possible, is rarely successful. Segmental resection can be attempted although care must be taken at the site of anastomosis during all subsequent procedures. If this is not possible then a controlled stoma can be considered as described below. NPWT has been used in the management of an entero-atmospheric fistula with good effect and may be described as the best option currently available, if used with caution. The principle goal of NPWT is to manage and divert the fistula output to prevent the spread of intra-abdominal sepsis [130-132]. Depending on the viscosity of the fistula output, drainage could be ineffective. To prevent this, a conduit from the source of the effluent through the dressing to the canister either by means of an ostomy bag or a drain can be considered [133]. Direct intubation of fistulas is not recommended. Visible fistulas can be managed by means of a floating stoma isolating the fistula with an ostomy bag. NPWT is often the only method available to achieve a secure bag adhesion, particularly in the mobile patient, and may simultaneously be used to manage the adjacent wound [133-135]. Remote fistulas are not suitable for direct stomal isolation. One option is to convert a remote entero-atmospheric fistula into an entero-cutaneous fistula by performing a separate incision and drainage. Once output is controlled and a granulating bed has been achieved, it may be possible to make conservative efforts to close by skin grafting [136]. NPWT may also protect skin from the fistula output thus helping to preserve the integrity of peri-wound skin [130, 137].

### *5) Management of Frozen Abdomen*

Prolonged inability to close the fascia will ultimately result in a 'fixed' abdomen for a diffuse granulation tissue in abdominal cavity and, hence, amongst the viscera. A risk factors for frozen abdomen in OA are represented by lack of wall closure within 10 days and non-use of plastic sheets over bowel loops. Once the abdominal wound has progressed to this phase, adhesions between the bowel loops and the fixity of bowel to abdominal wall

are so advanced, that attempts to release the adhesions by physical manipulation is highly likely to result in major lesions. At this stage, removal of all non-absorbable meshes is mandatory. Remaining available closure options involve a planned ventral hernia and include skin closure, secondary healing or split skin grafting. In this context, now that fascial closure is no longer possible, the main goal for application of NPWT could be to promote granulation tissue formation to create a suitable surface for rapid grafting. In fact, the degree of graft-take depends on the quality of the recipient wound bed, once granulation tissue has covered the surface of the exposed organs and a frozen abdominal wound is present [138, 139]. Under these circumstances the degree of adherence between the viscera and the abdominal wall is advanced and it does not allow application of the non-adherent interface layer. The granulation tissue and underlying organs are delicate and must be protected by the use of a wound contact layer placed between the NPWT wound filler and the wound bed. The wound contact layer prevents growth of newly formed granulation tissue into the foam NPWT wound filler which could be harmful for the risk of damage to the underlying tissue during dressing changes. In fact, a correlation has been reported between the number of cicles of NPWT
and fistula formation [140]. Once granulation tissue has formed over the surface of the bowel, particularly in large defects, split skin graft is the only option to rapidly close the abdomen [141-144].

***6) Sequential Dynamic Closure Technique Along with NPWT***

Any fascial closure should be 'tension free' in order to avoid ischemia and subsequent necrosis of the fascial and to reduce the risk of ACS. Sequential dynamic primary closure involves the sequential application of an increasing tension to the fascia, at each repeat exploration in order to eventually reach an early primary fascial closure. Application of dynamic suturing, also by mesh and/or particular devices [145-150], combined with NPWT seems to result in an overall fascial closure rate near to 80% [151]. Pliakos et al. [152], Burlew et al. [146] and Rasilainen et al. [153] independently reported significantly improved rates of fascial closure in patients who received NPWT in addition to dynamic closure compared with NPWT alone. This could mean that adoption of sequential closure with NPWT might extend the window during which fascial closure is possible. This would allow more time for resuscitation and sufficient recovery preserving anyway the option of fascial closure.

## Staged Abdominal Reconstruction

After DCS for trauma patients and during application of TAC system, when the patient has been adequately resuscitated as demonstrated by correction of hypothermia, acidosis, and coagulopathy, OA management must aim to a staged abdominal reconstruction (STAR). This can usually be accomplished within 36 hours. STAR serves three main functions: washout to reduce contamination and control intra-abdominal sepsis, resection or debridement of devitalized or contaminated tissue, and, especially, reconstruction of the gastrointestinal tract. It has been shown to improve the outcomes in severely injured trauma patients [154]. An ideal setting for reconstruction of internal injuries must be achieved [155, 156]. Injured devitalized tissue is resected, and gastrointestinal injuries can be anastomosed safely, mitigating the necessity for obligate ostomy. However, in high risk patients, ostomy remains the most conservative approach [157].

## Definitive Fascial Closure

### Timing

Once reconstruction phase is concluded and functional status of patient is not further dependent on cleanness and hemostasis of surgical field, the ultimate goal of surgeon is to achieve definitive fascial closure. Generally, early fascial closure is defined as a re-approximated closure of abdominal fascia within the window of 10 days an OA: it is easily achieved before the appearance of granulation tissue with simple suturing of fascial edges or by applying wall traction techniques [158, 159]. However, the abdominal viscera will become cocoon in the 14-day period to 21-day period and, commonly, after 10 days complications rate increases. As specified above, attempting to re-enter into the abdomen cavity to solve adhesions between viscera and abdominal wall to allow for an easier abdominal fascial closure is both difficult and dangerous. To improve survival rate and hospital service utilization, early fascial closure is routinely preferred to achieve a permanent abdominal closure, but it may not be feasible or prudent for specific patients with critical illness. In fact, a forced fascial closure in an early phase of OA may lead to intra-abdominal hypertension, possibly related to subsequent multiple organ dysfunction syndrome and additional re-laparotomies. Again, early fascial closure for patients with extensive abdominal wall defects would result in at least 50% recurrence rate of abdominal wound dehiscence [160].

When an early closure is impossible, delayed abdominal closure, achieved by absorbable or non-absorbable synthetic grafts as well as biological meshes, is an alternative reconstructive operation for the unclosed abdomen to be completed within 6–12 months or longer after OA [161-163].

However, in this case the surgeon is limited in the available surgical options: 1) bridge repair of the fascial defect using a mesh for a bridge closure; (2) abdominal wall reconstruction using most commonly a component separation procedure; 3) planned ventral hernia [164].

## Fascial Bridge

A fascial bridge closure may be considered in order to treat a persistent abdominal fascial defect after OA management. Fansler et al. [165] reported their experience with the fascial bridge closure of the OA with permanent prosthetic mesh. In a series of combined trauma and abdominal sepsis patients, polypropylene was used as a fascial bridge for definitive closure. They had significant complications including a 50% enterocutaneous fistula rate. Again. Voyles et al. [166] reported a similar experience with a high rate of complications and fistula formation. The association of synthetic prosthetic mesh with bacterial colonization is well known and, once infected, the prosthetic mesh becomes a chronic source of contamination. The use of permanent prosthetic (i.e., polypropylene, polytetrafluoroethylene, and polyester) has been abandoned in these situations because of the high rates of complications. From a decade biological mesh material has been commercially available. Biological meshes originate from human donors, bovine, and porcine animals and have been successfully used to bridge the abdominal wall defect. Human acellular dermal matrix (AlloDerm, LifeCell Corp.) has been shown to be successfully used as a fascial bridge after OA in multiple studies. It does not seem to form significant adhesions, to be negatively affected by bacterial contamination, and hence does not require removal in the setting of infection [167-173]. Once human acellular dermal matrix has developed a granulated tissue ground, a skin graft can be placed. Some authors noted that when no soft-tissue coverage is available, keeping the graft moist is critical to the graft's survival. NPWT is most often used for this purpose decreasing also bacterial colonization on the grafts. The long-term success of the use of biological material as a fascial bridge after OA is unclear. There are a number of studies suggesting that the long-term strength of this material decreases overtime. This effect may be attributable to collagen re-modeling, mesh attenuation, or tissue growth resulting in a high rate of hernia formation. However, bridge ventral hernia repairs with biological meshes have been performed after trauma and many patients have had definitive solutions [174].

## Acute Component Separation

One option for delayed closure of OA is an abdominal wall reconstruction using the component separation techniques. Ramirez et al. [175] were the first to describe the component separation technique for reconstruction of large abdominal wall fascial defect without the use of prosthetic mesh. The technique described 1) the anterior abdominal wall skin flaps developed and dissected out to the anterior superior iliac spine and the chest wall, 2) the aponeurosis of the external oblique muscle divided laterally to the semilunar line at the level of the xiphoid, 3) the external oblique dissected allowing the medial mobilization of the rectus myofascial component, and 4) the midline sutured together. The component separation, with its different versions, has become the most commonly used surgical technique for closure of large "planned" ventral hernias with a skin graft during the elective reconstructive phase [176-179]. Its use for definitive closure in the setting of an OA has not been well studied. Formal component separation is generally considered an "elective" reconstructive technique, because its use in the acute setting in the face of resolving intra-abdominal sepsis, visceral, and abdominal wall edema is not advisable.

## Planned Ventral Hernia

Once it has been determined that it is not possible to approximate the abdominal fascia, the planned ventral hernia technique is an option to consider for delayed closure of OA [180]. The initial goal of a planned ventral hernia is to keep the viscera within the abdominal cavity. This is accomplished by using an absorbable mesh to prevent evisceration. This allows time for the viscera to adhere together. Once the base of the open wound has granulated, a skin graft can be performed to cover the viscera. If the fascial defect is not large, another option is to elevate skin flaps and perform a skin only closure [181]. Caution must be exercised when elevating skin flaps in the setting of continued intra-abdominal sepsis, lack of source control, and massive visceral edema; because this setting has a high risk of skin flap infarction and flap loss. In this setting, allowing the wound base to progress to a good granulated base and proceeding to skin graft tissue coverage may be the safest option [176, 182].

## REFERENCES


[1] Ogilvie, WH. The late complications of abdominal war-wounds. *Lancet.*, 1940, 2, 253–256.

[2] Pringle, JH. Notes on the Arrest of Hepatic Hemorrhage Due to Trauma. *Ann Surg*, 1908, 48,541-9.

[3] Walt, AJ. The surgical management of hepatic trauma and its complications. Hunterian Lecture delivered at the Royal College of Surgeons of England. *Ann R Coll Surg Engl*, 1969, 45, 319–339.

[4] Rotondo, MF; Schwab, CW; McGonigal, MD; et al. 'Damage control': an approach for improved survival in exsanguinating penetrating abdominal injury. *J Trauma.*, 1993, 35, 375–382.

[5] Thorsen, K; Ringdal, KG; Strand, K; Søreide, E; Hagemo J; Søreide, K. Clinical and cellular effects of hypothermia, acidosis and coagulopathy in major injury. *Br J Surg.*, 2011 Jul, 98, 894-907.

[6] Duchesne, JC; McSwain, NE; Jr. Cotton, BA; Hunt, JP; Dellavolpe, J; Lafaro, K; et al. Damage control resuscitation: the new face of damage control. *J Trauma*, 2010, 69, 976–990.

[7] Rotondo, MF; Zonies, DH. The damage control sequence and underlying logic. *Surg Clin North Am*, 1997, 77, 761–777

[8] John, B; Kortbeek Saud, A. Al Turki American College of Surgeons Committee on Trauma. Advanced Trauma Life Support for Doctors. Students Course Manual (8th edn). *American College of Surgeons Committee on Trauma, Chicago*, 2004.

[9] Rossaint, R; Bouillon, B; Cerny, V; Coats, TJ; Duranteau, J; Fernandez-Mondejar, E; et al. Management of bleeding following major trauma: an updated European guideline. *Crit Care*, 2010, 14, R52.

[10] Søreide, E; Smith, CE. Hypothermia in trauma. In Trauma Anesthesia, Smith CE (ed). Cambridge University Press: Cambridge, 2008, 445–464.

[11] Jurkovich, GJ. Environmental cold-induced injury. *Surg Clin North Am*, 2007, 87, 247–267, viii.

[12] Tsuei, BJ; Kearney, PA. Hypothermia in the trauma patient. *Injury*, 2004, 35, 7–15.

[13] Hildebrand, F; Giannoudis, PV; van Griensven, M; Chawda, M; Pape, HC. Pathophysiologic changes and effects of hypothermia on outcome in elective surgery and trauma patients. *Am J Surg*, 2004, 187, 363–371.

[14] Danzl, DF; Pozos, RS. Accidental hypothermia. *N Engl J Med*, 1994, 331, 1756–1760.

[15] Biem, J; Koehncke, N; Classen, D; Dosman, J. Out of the cold: management of hypothermia and frostbite. *CMAJ*, 2003, 168, 305–311.

[16] Mallet, ML. Pathophysiology of accidental hypothermia. *QJM*, 2002, 95, 775–785.

[17] Kheirbek, T; Kochanek, AR; Alam, HB. Hypothermia in bleeding trauma: a friend or a foe? *Scand J Trauma Resusc Emerg Med*, 2009, 17, 65.

[18] Martini, WZ. Fibrinogen metabolic responses to trauma. *Scand J Trauma Resusc Emerg Med*, 2009, 17, 2.

[19] Hess, JR; Brohi, K; Dutton, RP; Hauser, CJ; Holcomb, JB; Kluger, Y; et al. The coagulopathy of trauma: a review of mechanisms. *J Trauma*, 2008, 65, 748–754.

[20] Inaba, K; Teixeira, PG; Rhee, P; Brown, C; Salim, A; DuBose, J; et al. Mortality impact of hypothermia after cavitary explorations in trauma. *World J Surg*, 2009, 33, 864–869.

[21] Martin, RS; Kilgo, PD; Miller, PR; Hoth, JJ; Meredith, JW; Chang, MC. Injury-associated hypothermia: an analysis of the 2004 National Trauma Data Bank. *Shock*, 2005, 24, 114–118.

[22] Wang, HE; Callaway, CW; Peitzman, AB; Tisherman, SA. Admission hypothermia and outcome after major trauma. *Crit Care Med*, 2005, 33, 1296–1301.

[23] Aitken, LM; Hendrikz, JK; Dulhunty, JM; Rudd, MJ. Hypothermia and associated outcomes in seriously injured trauma patients in a predominantly sub-tropical climate. *Resuscitation*, 2009, 80, 217–223.

[24] Shafi, S; Elliott, AC; Gentilello, L. Is hypothermia simply a marker of shock and injury severity or an independent risk factor for mortality in trauma patients? Analysis of a large national trauma registry. *J Trauma*, 2005, 59, 1081–1085.

[25] Bernabei, AF; Levison, MA; Bender, JS. The effects of hypothermia and injury severity on blood loss during trauma laparotomy. *J Trauma*, 1992, 33, 835–839.

[26] Jurkovich, GJ; Greiser, WB; Luterman, A; Curreri, PW. Hypothermia in trauma victims: an ominous predictor of survival. *J Trauma*, 1987, 27, 1019–1024.

[27] Gentilello, LM; Jurkovich, GJ; Stark, MS; Hassantash, SA; O'Keefe, GE. Is hypothermia in the victim of major trauma protective or harmful? A randomized, prospective study. *Ann Surg*, 1997, 226, 439–447.

[28] Zehtabchi, S; Soghoian, S; Sinert, R. Utility of Stewart's strong ion difference as a predictor of major injury after trauma in the ED. *Am J Emerg Med*, 2007, 25, 938–941.

[29] Jones, RC; Yost, MJ; Fann, SA. Cocaine induced acidosis in the trauma patient: a potential confounding factor. *Am Surg*, 2008, 74, 1125–1127.

[30] Funk, GC; Doberer, D; Kneidinger, N; Lindner, G; Holzinger, U; Schneeweiss, B. Acid–base disturbances in critically ill patients with cirrhosis. *Liver Int*, 2007, 27, 901–909.

[31] Dirkmann, D; Hanke, AA; G¨ orlinger, K; Peters, J. Hypothermia and acidosis synergistically impair coagulation in human whole blood. *Anesth Analg*, 2008, 106, 1627–1632.

[32] Engstrom, M; Schott, U; Romner, B; Reinstrup, P. Acidosis impairs the coagulation: a thromboelastographic study. *J Trauma*, 2006, 61, 624–628.

[33] Hess, JR; Holcomb, JB; Hoyt, DB. Damage control resuscitation: the need for specific blood products to treat the coagulopathy of trauma. *Transfusion*, 2006, 46, 685–686.

[34] Martini, WZ; Holcomb, JB. Acidosis and coagulopathy: the differential effects on fibrinogen synthesis and breakdown in pigs. *Ann Surg*, 2007, 246, 831–835.

[35] Martini, WZ. Coagulopathy by hypothermia and acidosis: mechanisms of thrombin generation and fibrinogen availability. *J Trauma*, 2009, 67, 202–208.

[36] Davis, JW; Parks, SN; Kaups, KL; Gladen, HE; O'Donnell-Nicol, S. Admission base deficit predicts transfusion requirements and risk of complications. *J Trauma*, 1996, 41, 769–774.

[37] Blow, O; Magliore, L; Claridge, JA; Butler, K; Young, JS. The golden hour and the silver day: detection and correction of occult hypoperfusion within 24 hours improves outcome from major trauma. *J Trauma*, 1999, 47, 964–969.

[38] Thom, O; Taylor, DM;Wolfe, RE; Myles, P; Krum, H; Wolfe, R. Pilot study of the prevalence, outcomes and detection of occult hypoperfusion in trauma patients. *Emerg Med J*, 2010, 27, 470–472.

[39] Tieu, BH; Holcomb, JB; Schreiber, MA. Coagulopathy: its pathophysiology and treatment in the injured patient. *World J Surg*, 2007, 31, 1055–1064.

[40] Hoyt, DB. Blood and war – lest we forget. *J Am Coll Surg*, 2009, 209, 681–686.

[41] Levy, JH; Dutton, RP; Hemphill, JC; III, Shander, A; Cooper, D; Paidas, MJ; et al. Hemostasis Summit Participants. Multidisciplinary approach to the challenge of hemostasis. *Anesth Analg*, 2010, 110, 354–364.

[42] Brohi, K; Cohen, MJ; Ganter, MT; Schultz, MJ; Levi, M; Mackersie, RC; et al. Acute coagulopathy of trauma: hypoperfusion induces systemic anticoagulation and hyperfibrinolysis. *J Trauma*, 2008, 64, 1211–1217.

[43] MacLeod, JB. Trauma and coagulopathy: a new paradigm to consider. *Arch Surg*, 2008, 143, 797–801.

[44] Brohi, K; Cohen, MJ; Ganter, MT; Matthay, MA; Mackersie, RC; Pittet, JF. Acute traumatic coagulopathy: initiated by hypoperfusion: modulated through the protein C pathway? *Ann Surg*, 2007, 245, 812–818.

[45] Davenport, RA; Brohi, K. Coagulopathy in trauma patients: importance of thrombocyte function? *Curr Opin Anaesthesiol*, 2009, 22, 261–266.

[46] MacLeod, JB; Lynn, M; McKenney, MG; Cohn, SM; Murtha, M. Early coagulopathy predicts mortality in trauma. *J Trauma*, 2003, 55, 39–44.

[47] Brohi, K; Singh, J; Heron, M; Coats, T. Acute traumatic coagulopathy. *J Trauma*, 2003, 54, 1127–1130.

[48] Chaudry, IH; Bland, KI. Cellular mechanisms of injury after major trauma. *Br J Surg*, 2009, 96, 1097–1098.

[49] Chesebro, BB; Rahn, P; Carles, M; Esmon, CT; Xu, J; Brohi, K; et al. Increase in activated protein C mediates acute traumatic coagulopathy in mice. *Shock*, 2009, 32, 659–665.

[50] Cohen, MJ; Bir, N; Rahn, P; Dotson, R; Brohi, K; Chesebro, BB; et al. Protein C depletion early after trauma increases the risk of ventilator-associated pneumonia. *J Trauma*, 2009, 67, 1176–1181.

[51] Gando, S. Acute coagulopathy of trauma shock and coagulopathy of trauma: a rebuttal. You are now going down the wrong path. *J Trauma*, 2009, 67, 381–383.

[52] Johansson, PI; Ostrowski, SR; Secher, NH. Management of major blood loss: an update. *Acta Anaesthesiol Scand*, 2010, 54, 1039–1049.

[53] Johansson, PI; Stissing, T; Bochsen, L; Ostrowski, SR; Thrombelastography and thromboelastometry in assessing coagulopathy in trauma. *Scand J Trauma Resusc Emerg Med*, 2009, 17, 45.

[54] Ganter, MT; Hofer, CK. Coagulation monitoring: current techniques and clinical use of viscoelastic point-of-care coagulation devices. *Anesth Analg*, 2008, 106, 1366–1375.

[55] Jacoby, RC; Owings, JT; Holmes, J; Battistella, FD; Gosselin, RC; Paglieroni, TG. Platelet activation and function after trauma. *J Trauma*, 2001, 51, 639–647.

[56] Phan, HH; Wisner, DH. Should we increase the ratio of plasma/platelets to red blood cells in massive transfusion: what is the evidence? ; *Vox Sang*, 2010, 98, 395–402.

[57] Mitra, B; Mori, A; Cameron, PA; Fitzgerald, M; Paul, E; Street, A. Fresh frozen plasma (FFP) use during massive blood transfusion in trauma resuscitation. *Injury*, 2010, 41, 35–39.

[58] Greer, SE; Rhynhart, KK; Gupta, R; Corwin, HL. New developments in massive transfusion in trauma. *Curr Opin Anaesthesiol*, 2010, 23, 246–250.

[59] Schochl, H; Frietsch, T; Pavelka, M; Jambor, C. Hyperfibrinolysis after major trauma: differential diagnosis of lysis patterns and prognostic value of thrombelastometry. *J Trauma*, 2009, 67, 125–131.

[60] Kashuk, JL; Moore, EE; Sawyer, M; Wohlauer, M; Pezold, M; Barnett, C; et al. Primary fibrinolysis is integral in the pathogenesis of the acute coagulopathy of trauma. *Ann Surg*, 2010, 252, 434–444.

[61] Cosgriff, N; Moore, EE; Sauaia, A; Kenny-Moynihan, M; Burch, JM; Galloway, B. Predicting life-threatening coagulopathy in the massively transfused trauma patient: hypothermia and acidoses revisited. *J Trauma*, 1997, 42, 857–861.

[62] Kron, IL; Harmon, PK; Nolan, SP; (1984). The measurement of intra-abdominal pressure as a criterion for abdominal re-exploration. *Ann Surg*, 1984, 199, 28–30

[63] Baggot, MG. Abdominal blow-out: a concept. *Anesth Analg*, 1951, 30, 295-9.

[64] Harman, PK; Kron, IL; McLachlan, HD; Freedlender, AE; Nolan, SP. Elevated intra-abdominal pressure and renal function. *Ann Surg*, 1982, 196, 594-7

[65] Richards, WO; Scovil, W; Shin, B; Reed, W. Acute renal failure associated with increased intra-abdominal pressure. *Ann Surg*, 1983, 197, 183-7.

[66] Sugrue, M; Buist, MD; Hourihan, F; Deane, S; Bauman, A; Hillman, K. Prospective study of intra-abdominal hypertension and renal function after laparotomy. *Br Surg*, 1995, 82, 235-8.
[67] Doty, JM; Saggi, BH; Blocher, CR; Fakhry, I; Gehr, T; Sica, D; et al. Effects of increate renal parenchymal pressure on renal function. *Trauma*, 2000, 48, 874-7.
[68] Doty, JM; Saggi, BH; Sugerman, HJ; Blocher, CR; Pin, R; Fakhry, I; et al. Effect of increate renal venous pressure on renal function. *Trauma*, 1999, 47, 1000-3.
[69] Iberti, TJ; Kelly, KM; Gentili, DR; Hirsch, S; Benjamin, E. A simple technique to accurately determine intra-abdominal pressure. *Crit Care Med*, 1987, 15, 1140-2.
[70] Cullen, DJ; Coyle, JP; Teplich, R; Long, MC. Cardiovascular, pulmonary, and renal effects of massively increased intra-abdominal pressure in critically ill patients. *Crit Care Med*, 1989, 17, 118-21
[71] Fietsam, R; Jr. Villalba, M; Glover, HL; Clark, K. Intra-abdominal compartment syndrome as a complication of ruptured abdominal aortic aneurysm repair. *Am Surg*, 1989, 55, 396-402.
[72] DuBose, JJ; Scalea, T; Holcomb, JB; et al. Open abdominal management after damage-control laparotomy for trauma: a prospective observational American Association for the Surgery of Trauma multicenter study. *J Trauma Acute Care Surg.*, 2013, 74, 113-122.
[73] Regner, JL; Kobayashi, L; Coimbra, R. Surgical Strategies for Management of the Open Abdomen. *World J Surg*, 2012, 36, 497–510
[74] Diaz, JJ; Jr. Cullinane, DC; Dutton, WD; et al. The management of the open abdomen in trauma and emergency general surgery: Part 1—Damage Control. *J Trauma.*, 2010, 68, 1425–1438
[75] Teixeira, PGR; Salim, A; Inaba, K; et al. A prospective look at the current state of open abdomens. *Am Surg*, 2008, 74, 891-897
[76] Schein, M; Paul, N. Rogers. Schein's Common Sense Emergency Abdominal, An Unconventional Book for Trainees and Thinking Surgeons. 3th Edition. *USA, Springer*, 2009
[77] Björck, M1; Bruhin, A; Cheatham, M; Hinck, D; Kaplan, M; Manca, G; Wild, T; Windsor, A. Classification--important step to improve management of patients with an open abdomen. *World J Surg.*, 2009, 33, 1154-7.
[78] Boele van Hensbroek, P1; Wind, J; Dijkgraaf, MG; Busch, OR; Goslings, JC. Temporary closure of the open abdomen: a

systematic review on delayed primary fascial closure in patients with an open abdomen. *World J Surg.*, 2009 Feb, 33,199-207

[79] Cuesta, MA; Doblas, M; Castaneda, L; Bengoechea, E. Sequential abdominal reexploration with the zipper technique. *World J Surg*, 1991, 15,74–80

[80] Doyon, A; Devroede, G. Viens Det al. Asimple, inexpensive, life-saving way to perform iterative laparotomy in patients with severe intra-abdominal sepsis. *Colorectal Dis*, 2001, 3, 115–121

[81] Howdieshell, TR; Proctor, CD; Sternberg, E; Cue, JI; Mondy, JS; Hawkins, ML. Temporary abdominal closure followed by definitive abdominal wall reconstruction of the open abdomen. *Am J Surg*, 2004, 188, 301–306

[82] Smith, PC; Tweddell, JS; Bessey, PQ. Alternative approaches to abdominal wound closure in severely injured patients with massive visceral edema. *J Trauma*, 1992, 32, 16–20

[83] Suliburk, JW; Ware, DN; Balogh, Z; et al. Vacuum-assisted wound closure achieves early fascial closure of open abdomens after severe trauma. *J Trauma*, 2003, 55, 1155–1160

[84] Tremblay, LN; Feliciano, DV; Schmidt, J; et al. Skin only or silo closure in the critically ill patient with an open abdomen. *Am J Surg*, 2001, 182, 670–675

[85] Barker, DE; Kaufman, HJ; Smith, LA; Ciraulo, DL; Richart, CL; Burns, RP. Vacuum pack technique of temporary abdominal closure: a 7-year experience with 112 patients. *J Trauma*, 2000, 48, 201–206

[86] Cipolla, J; Stawicki, SP; Hoff, WS; et al. A proposed algorithm for managing the open abdomen. *Am Surg*, 2005, 71, 202-207

[87] Keramati, M; Srivastava, A; Sakabu, S; et al. The Wittmann PatchTM as a temporary abdominal closure device after decompressive celiotomy for abdominal compartment syndrome following burn. *Burns*, 2008, 34, 493–497

[88] Olona, C; Caro, A; Duque, E; et al. Comparative study of open abdomen treatment: ABTheraTM vs. abdominal dressingTM . *Hernia.*, 2015, 19, 323-8.

[89] Navsaria, PH; Bunting, M; Omoshoro-James, J; et al. Temporary closure of open abdominal wounds by modified sandwich-vacuum pack technique. *Br J Surg*, 2003, 90, 718-722

[90] Miller, PR; Meredith, JW; Johnson, JC; et al. Prospective evaluation of vacuum-assisted fascial closure after open abdomen planned ventral hernia rate is substantially reduced. *Ann Surg*, 2004, 239, 608–616

[91] Roberts, DJ; Zygun, DA; Grendar, J; et al. Negative-pressure wound therapy for critically ill adults with open abdominal wounds: a systematic review. *J Trauma Acute Care Surg.*, 2012, 73, 629-639

[92] Rycerz, AM; Slack, P; McNulty, AK. Distribution assessment comparing continuous and periodic wound instillation in conjunction with negative pressure wound therapy using an agar-based model. *Int Wound J*, 2013, 10, 214–220

[93] Sherck, J; Seiver, A; Shatney, C; et al. Covering the open abdomen: the better technique. *Am Surg*, 1998, 64(9), 854-857.

[94] Rycerz, AM; Allen, D; Lessing, MC. Science supporting negative pressure wound therapy with instillation. *International Wound Journal*, 2013, 10, 20–24

[95] Campbell, AM; Khun, WP; Barker, P. Vacuum-assisted closure of the open abdomen in a resource-limited setting. *SAJS*, 2010, 48,114-115

[96] Campbell, A; Chang, M; Fabian, T; Franz, M; Kaplan, M; Moore, F; Reed, RL; Scott, B; Silverman, R. Open Abdomen Advisory Panel: management of the open abdomen: from initial operation to definitive closure. *Am Surg*, 2009, 75, S1-S22

[97] Brock, WB1; Barker, DE; Burns, RP. Temporary closure of open abdominal wounds: the vacuum pack. Brock WB1, Barker DE, Burns RP. *Am Surg.*, 1995 Jan, 61, 30-5.

[98] Duff, JH; Moffat, J. Abdominal sepsis managed by leaving abdomen open. *Surgery*, 1981, 90, 774–78

[99] Schein, M; Saadia, R; Jamieson, JR; Decker, GA. The "sandwich technique" in the management of the open abdomen. *Br J Surg*, 1986, 73, 369–70

[100] Boele van Hensbroek, P; Wind, J; Dijkgraaf, MGW; et al. Temporary closure of the open abdomen: a systematic review on delayed primary fascial closure in patients with an open abdomen. *World J Surg*, 2009, 33, 199–207

[101] Garner, GB1; Ware, DN; Cocanour, CS; Duke, JH; McKinley, BA; Kozar, RA; Moore, FA. Vacuum-assisted wound closure provides early fascial reapproximation in trauma patients with open abdomens. *Am J Surg.*, 2001 Dec, 182, 630-8.

[102] Miller, PR; Thompson, JT; Faler, BJ; et al. Late fascial closure in lieu of ventral hernia: the next step in open abdomen management. *J Trauma*, 2002, 53, 843–49

[103] Miller, PR; Meredith, JW; Johnson, JC; Chang, MC. Prospective Evaluation of Vacuum-Assisted Fascial Closure After Open Abdomen. *Ann Surg*, 2004, 239, 608–16

[104] Barbara Elize Kreis, Johan Coenraad, Alexander, de Mol van Otterloo, Robert Walter Kreis. Open abdomen management: A review of its history and a proposed management algorithm. *Med Sci Monit*, 2013, 19, 524-533

[105] Bruhin, A; Ferreira, F; Charikerc, M; Smith, J; Runkel, N. Systematic review and evidence based recommendations for the use of Negative Pressure Wound Therapy in the open abdomen. *International Journal of Surgery*, 2014, 12, 1105-1114

[106] Orgill, DP; Manders, EK; Sumpio, BE; et al. The mechanism of action of vacuum assisted closure: more to learn. *Surgery.*, 2009, 146, 40-51.

[107] Huang, C; Leavitt, T; Bayer, LR; Orgill, DP. Effect of negative pressure wound therapy on wound healing. *Curr Probl Surg.*, 2014, 51, 301-31.

[108] Dubose, JJ; Lundy, JB. Enterocutaneous fistulas in the setting of trauma and critical illness. *Clin Colon Rectal Surg.*, 2010, 23, 182-9.

[109] Batacchi, S; Matano, S; Nella, A; et al. Vacuum-assisted closure device enhances recovery of critically ill patients following emergency surgical procedures. *Crit Care.*, 2009, 13, R194

[110] Kubiak, BD; Albert, SP; Gatto, LA; et al. Peritoneal negative pressure therapy prevents multiple organ injury in a chronic porcine sepsis and ischemia/reperfusion model. *Shock vol.*, 34 2010, 5, 525–534.

[111] Hatch, QM; Osterhout, LM; Ashraf, A; Podbielski, J; Kozar, RA; Wade, CE; Holcomb, JB; Cotton, BA. Current use of damage-control laparotomy, closure rates, and predictors of early fascial closure at the first take-back. *J Trauma.*, 2011, 70, 1429, 1436.

[112] Barker, DE; Green, JM; Maxwell, R; et al. Experience with vacuum-pack temporary abdominal wound closure in 258 trauma and general and vascular surgical patients, *J. Am. Coll. Surg.*, 2007, 204, 784 792.

[113] Condè Green, A; Chung, ATL; Holton, LH; et al. Incisional negative-pressure wound therapy versus conventional dressings following abdominal wall reconstruction: a comparative study, *Ann. Plast. Surg.*, 2012, 71, 394 397.

[114] Vargo, D. Negative pressure wound therapy in the prevention of wound infection in high risk abdominal wound closures, *Am. J. Surg.*, 2012, 204, 1021 1023.

[115] Blackham, AU; Farrah, JP; McCoy, TP; et al. Prevention of surgical site infections in high-risk patients with laparotomy incisions using negative pressure therapy, *Am. J. Surg*., 2013, 205, 647-654.

[116] Stannard, JP; Volgas, DA; McGwin, G; et al. Incisional negative pressure wound therapy after high-risk lower extremity fractures, *J. Orthop. Trauma*, 2012, 26, 37-42.

[117] Stannard, JP; Robinson, JT; Anderson, ER; et al. Negative pressure wound therapy to treat hematomas and surgical incisions following high-energy trauma, *J. Trauma*, 2006, 60, 1301-1306.

[118] Reddix, RN; Leng, XI; Woodall, J; et al. The effect of incisional negative pressure therapy on wound complications after acetabular fracture surgery, *J. Surg. Orthop. Adv*., 2010, 19, 91-97.

[119] Schmedes, GW; Banks, CA; Malin, BT; et al. Massive flap donor sites and the role of negative pressure wound therapy, Otolaryngol. *Head Neck Surg*., 2012, 147, 1049-1053.

[120] Masden, D; Goldstein, J; Endara, M; et al. Negative pressure wound therapy for at-risk surgical closures in patients with multiple comorbidities: a prospective randomized controlled study, *Ann. Surg*., 2012, 255, 1043-1047.

[121] Friese, RS. The open abdomen: definitions, management principles, and nutrition support considerations. *Nutr Clin Pract*, 2012, 27, 492-498

[122] Burlew, CC; Moore, EE; Cuschieri, J; et al. Who should we feed? A Western Trauma Associationmulti-institutional study of enteral nutrition in the open abdomen after injury. *J Trauma Acute Care Surg*, 2012, 73,1380-1388

[123] Byrnes, MC; Reicks, P; Irwin, E. Early enteral nutrition can be successfully implemented in trauma patients with an "open abdomen." *Am J Surg*, 2010,199, 359–363

[124] Majercik, S; Kinikini, M; White, T. Enteroatmospheric fistula: from soup to nuts. *Nutr Clin Pract*, 2012, 27, 507-512

[125] Polk, TM; Schwab, CW. Metabolic and nutritional support of the enterocutaneous fistula patient: a three-phase approach. *World J Surg*, 2012, 36, 524–533

[126] Yuan, Y; Ren, J; Gu, G; et al. Early enteral nutrition improves outcomes of open abdomen in gastrointestinal fistula patients complicated with severe sepsis. *Nutr Clin Pract*, 2011, 26, 688-94.

[127] Draus, JM; Jr. Huss, SA; Harty, NJ; Cheadle, WG; Larson, GM. Enterocutaneous fistula: are treatments improving? *Surgery*., 2006, 140, 570 –576.

[128] Hollender, LF; Meyer, C; Avet, D; Zeyer, B. Postoperative fistulas of the small intestine: therapeutic principles. *World J Surg.*, 1983, 7, 474 – 480.

[129] Dudrick, SJ; Maharaj, AR; McKelvey, AA. Artificial nutritional support in patients with gastrointestinal fistulas. *World J Surg.*, 1999, 23, 570 – 576.

[130] Al-Khoury, G; Kaufman, D; Hirshberg, A. Improved control of exposed fistula in the open abdomen, *J. Am. Coll. Surg.*, 2008, 206, 397, 398.

[131] Stremitzer, S; Dal Borgo, A; Wild, T; et al., Successful bridging treatment and healing of enteric fistulae by vacuum-assisted closure (VAC) therapy and targeted drainage in patients with open abdomen, *Int. J. Colorectal Dis.*, 2011, 26, 661-666.

[132] Marinis, A; Gkiokas, G; Anastasopoulos, G; et al. Surgical techniques for the management of enteroatmospheric fistulae, Surg. Infect. *Larchmt*, 2009, 10, 47, 52.

[133] Goverman, J; Yelon, J; Platz, JJ; et al. The "Fistula VAC," a technique for management of enterocutaneous fistulae arising within the open abdomen: report of 5 cases, *J. Trauma*, 2006, 60, 428,431.

[134] Draus, JM; Huss, S; Harty, NJ; et al. Enterocutaneous fistula: are treatments improving? *Surgery*, 2006, 140, 570, 576.

[135] Banasiewicz, T; Borejsza-Wysocki, M; Meissner, W; et al. Topical negative pressure as a safe and helpful treatment in patients with large abdominal wounds with multiple fistulae, *Colorectal Dis.*, 2010, 12, 1166, 1167.

[136] Byrnes, MC; Riggle, A; Beilman, G; et al., A novel technique to skin graft abdominal wall wounds surrounding enterocutaneous fistulas, Surg. Infect. *Larchmt*, 2010, 11, 505, 509.

[137] Cro, C; George, KJ; Donnelly, J; Irwin, ST; Gardiner, KR. Vacuum assisted closure system in the management of enterocutaneous fistulae, *Postgrad. Med. J.*, 2002, 78, 364, 365.

[138] Shaikh, I; Ballard-Wilson, A; Yalamarthi, S; et al., Use of topical negative pressure in assisted abdominal closure does not lead to high incidence of enteric fistulae, *Colorectal Dis.*, 2010, 12, 931, 934.

[139] Amin, AI; Shaikh, IA. Topical negative pressure in managing severe peritonitis: a positive contribution? *World J. Gastroenterol.*, 2009, 15, 3394, 3397.

[140] Schmelzle, M; Alldinger, I; Matthaei, H; et al. Long-term vacuum-assisted closure in open abdomen due to secondary peritonitis: a

retrospective evaluation of a selected group of patients, *Dig. Surg.*, 2010, 27, 272, 278.

[141] Vuerstaek, JD; Vainas, T; Wuite, J; et al. State-of-the-art treatment of chronic leg ulcers: a randomized controlled trial comparing vacuum-assisted closure (V.A.C.) with modern wound dressings, *J. Vasc. Surg.*, 2006, 44, 1029, 1037.

[142] Llanos, S; Danilla, S; Barraza, C; et al., Effectiveness of negative pressure closure in the integration of split thickness skin grafts: a randomized, double-masked, controlled trial, *Ann. Surg.*, 2006, 244, 700, 705.

[143] Korber, A; Franckson, T; Grabbe, S; et al. Vacuum assisted closure device improves the take of mesh grafts in chronic leg ulcer patients, *Dermatology*, 2008, 216, 250, 256.

[144] Vidrine, DM; Kaler, S; Rosenthal, EL. A comparison of negative-pressure dressings versus Bolster and splinting of the radial forearm donor site, Otolaryngol. *Head Neck Surg.*, 2005, 133, 403, 406.

[145] Kafka-Ritsch, R; Zitt, M; Schorn, N; et al., Open abdomen treatment with dynamic sutures and topical negative pressure resulting in a high primary fascia closure rate, *World J. Surg.*, 2012, 36, 1765, 1771.

[146] Burlew, CC; Moore, EE; Biffl, WL; et al. One hundred percent fascial approximation can be achieved in the postinjury open abdomen with a sequential closure protocol, *J. Trauma Acute Care Surg.*, 2012, 72, 235, 241.

[147] Sorelius, K; Wanhainen, A; Acosta, S; et al. Open abdomen treatment after aortic aneurysm repair with vacuum-assisted wound closure and meshmediated fascial traction. *Eur. J. Vasc. Endovasc. Surg.*, 2013, 45, 588-94.

[148] Kleif, J; Fabricius, R; Bertelsen, CA; et al. Promising results after vacuumassisted wound closure and mesh-mediated fascial traction, *Dan. Med. J.*, 2012, 59, A4495.

[149] Verdam, FJ; Dolmans, DE; Loos, MJ; et al. Delayed primary closure of the septic open abdomen with a dynamic closure system, *World J. Surg.*, 2011, 35, 2348, 2355.

[150] Salman, E; Yetis, F; Aksoy, M; et al. Use of dynamic wound closure system in conjunction with vacuum-assisted closure therapy in delayed closure of open abdomen, *Hernia*, 2014, 18, 99-104.

[151] Jose, J; Diaz, Jr. MD; Daniel, C; Cullinane, Nicole Stassen, MD; Eleanor, S; Winston, MD. The Management of the Open Abdomen in

Trauma andEmergency General Surgery: Part 1—Damage Control. *J Trauma.*, 2010, 68, 1425–1438.

[152] Pliakos, Papavramidis, TS; Mihalopoulos, N; et al. Vacuum-assisted closure in severe abdominal sepsis with or without retention sutured sequential fascial closure: a clinical trial, *Surgery*, 2010, 148, 947, 953.

[153] Rasilainen, SK; Mentula, PJ; Lepp€aniemi, AK. Vacuum and mesh-mediated fascial traction for primary closure of the open abdomen in critically ill surgical patients, *Br. J. Surg.*, 2012, 99, 1725, 1732.

[154] Hirshberg, A; Wall, MJ; Jr. Mattox, KL. Planned reoperation for trauma: a two year experience with 124 consecutive patients. *J Trauma.*, 1994, 37, 365–369.

[155] Ozguc, H; Yilmazlar, T; Gurluler, E; Ozen, Y; Korun, N; Zorluog˘lu, A. Staged abdominal repair in the treatment of intra-abdominal infection: analysis of 102 patients. *J Gastrointest Surg.*, 2003, 7, 646–651.

[156] Holzheimer, RG; Gathof, B. Re-operation for complicated secondary peritonitis—how to identify patients at risk for persistent sepsis. *Eur J Med Res.*, 2003, 8, 125–134.

[157] Finlay, IG; Edwards, TJ; Lambert, AW. Damage control laparotomy. *Br J Surg.*, 2004, 91, 83– 85.

[158] Kreis, BE; de Mol van Otterloo, EJ; Kreis, RW. Open abdomen management: a review of its history and a proposed management algorithm. *Med Sci Monit*, 2013, 19, 524-533

[159] Dennis, A; Vizinas, TA; Joseph, K; et al. Not so fast to skin graft: transabdominal wall traction closes most "domain loss" abdomens in the acute setting. *J Trauma Acute Care Surg.*, 2013, 74,1486-1492

[160] Paul, A; Korenkov, M; Peters, S; K¨ohler, L; Fischer, S; Troidl; H. Unacceptable results of the Mayo procedure for repair of abdominal incisional hernias. *European Journal of Surgery*, 1998, vol. 164, no. 5, 361–367,

[161] Campbell, A; Chang, M; Fabian, T; et al. "Management of the open abdomen: from initial operation to definitive closure," *The American Surgeon*, 2009 vol. 75, supplement, 11, S1–S22.

[162] Cipolla, J; Stawicki, SP; S.Hoff, W; et al. "A proposed algorithm for managing the open abdomen," *The American Surgeon*, 2005, vol. 71, no. 3, 202–207.

[163] Schecter, WP; Ivatury, RR; Rotondo, MF; et al. Open abdomen after trauma and abdominal sepsis: a strategy for management, *J. Am. Coll. Surg.*, 2006, 203, 390, 396.

[164] Jose, J; Diaz, Jr. MD; William, D; Dutton, MD; Mickey, M; William, P; Riordan, MD; Christopher, D; Wohltmann, MD. Eastern Association for the Surgery of Trauma: A Review of the Management of the Open Abdomen—Part 2 "Management of the Open Abdomen." The Journal of TRAUMA Injury, Infection, and Critical Care, Volume 71, Number 2, August 2011

[165] Fansler, RF; Taheri, P; Cullinane, C; Sabates, B; Flint, LM. Polypropylene mesh closure of the complicated abdominal wound. *Am J Surg.*, 1995, 170, 15–18.

[166] Voyles, CR; Richardson, JD; Bland, KI; Tobin, GR; Flint, LM; Polk, HC; Jr. Emergency abdominal wall reconstruction with polypropylene mesh: short-term benefits versus long-term complications. *Ann Surg.*, 1981, 194, 219–223.

[167] Guy, JS; Miller, R; Morris, JA; Jr. Diaz, J; May, A. Early one-stage closure in patients with abdominal compartment syndrome: fascial replacement with human a cellular dermis and bi pedicle flaps. *Am Surg.*, 2003, 69, 1025–1028.

[168] Singh, MK; Rocca, JP; Rochon, C; Facciuto, ME; Sheiner, PA; Rodriguez- Davalos, MI. Open abdomen management with human acellular dermal matrix in liver transplant recipients. *Transplant Proc.*, 2008, 40, 3541– 3544.

[169] Taner, T; Cima, RR; Larson, DW; Dozois, EJ; Pemberton, JH; Wolff, BG. The use of human a cellular dermal matrix for para stomal hernia repair in patients with inflammatory bowel disease: a novel technique to repair fascial defects. *Dis Colon Rectum.*, 2009, 52, 349 –354.

[170] Liu, L; Li, JS; Li, N; Ren, JA; Zhao, YZ. Reconstruction of infected complex abdominal wall defects with auto genous pedicled demucosalized small intestinal sheet. *Surgery.*, 2009, 145, 114 –119.

[171] Diaz, JJ; Jr. Conquest, AM; Ferzoco, SJ; et al. Multi-institutional experience using human acellular dermal matrix for ventral hernia repair in a compromised surgical field. *Arch Surg.*, 2009, 144, 209 –215.

[172] Patton, JH; Jr. Berry, S; Kralovich, KA. Use of human acellular dermal matrix in complex and contaminated abdominal wall reconstructions. *Am J Surg.*, 2007, 193, 360 –363.

[173] Awad, SS; Rao, RK; Berger, DH; Albo, D; Bellows, CF. Microbiology of infected acellular dermal matrix (AlloDerm) in patients requiring complex abdominal closure after emergency surgery. *Surg Infect (Larchmt).*, 2009, 10, 79–84.

[174] Jin, J; Rosen, MJ; Blatnik, J; et al. Use of acellular dermal matrix for complicated ventral hernia repair: does technique affect outcomes? *J Am Coll Surg.*, 2007, 205, 654–660.
[175] Ramirez, OM; Ruas, E; Dellon, AL. "Components separation" method for closure of abdominal-wall defects: an anatomic and clinical study. *Plast Reconstr Surg.*, 1990, 86, 519 –526.
[176] Howdieshell, TR; Proctor, CD; Sternberg, E; Cue, JI; Mondy, JS; Hawkins, ML. Temporary abdominal closure followed by definitive abdominal wall reconstruction of the open abdomen. *Am J Surg.*, 2004, 188, 301– 306.
[177] Rodriguez, ED; Bluebond-Langner, R; Silverman, RP; et al. Abdominal wall reconstruction following severe loss of domain: the R Adams Cowley Shock Trauma Center algorithm. *Plast Reconstr Surg.*, 2007, 120, 669–680.
[178] Vargo, D. Component separation in the management of the difficult abdominal wall. *Am J Surg.*, 2004, 188, 633– 637.
[179] Kushimoto, S; Yamamoto, Y; Aiboshi, J; et al. Usefulness of the bilateral anterior rectus abdominis sheath turnover flap method for early fascial closure in patients requiring open abdominal management. *World J Surg.*, 2007, 31, 2– 8.
[180] Jernigan, TW; Fabian, TC; Croce, MA; et al. Staged management of giant abdominal wall defects: acute and long-term results. *Ann Surg.*, 2003, 238, 349 –355.
[181] Mathes, SJ; Steinwald, PM; Foster, RD; Hoffman, WY; Anthony, JP. Complex abdominal wall reconstruction: a comparison of flap and mesh closure. *Ann Surg.*, 2000, 232, 586 –596.
[182] Cohen, M; Morales, R; Jr. Fildes, J; Barrett, J. Staged reconstruction after gunshot wounds to the abdomen. *Plast Reconstr Surg.*, 2001, 108, 83–92.

In: Abdominal Trauma ...
Editor: Louise Santiago

ISBN: 978-1-63483-482-7


*Chapter 3*

# BACTERIAL PERITONITIS AND INTRA-ABDOMINAL ABSCESSES POST ABDOMINAL TRAUMA: ETIOLOGY AND ANTIMICROBIAL THERAPY IN THE ERA OF MULTI-DRUG RESISTANCE

***Wen-Liang Yu*[*] *and Khee-Siang Chan***
Department of Intensive Care Medicine, Chi Mei Medical Center, Tainan City, Taiwan

## ABSTRACT

Bacterial peritonitis and intra-abdominal abscesses are major complicated intra-abdominal infections post abdominal trauma. These infections are often associated with intestinal or mesenteric ischemic injury, hollow organ gangrene or perforation, intra-abdominal visceral laceration, infarction or perforation, severe pancreatitis, penetrating injury and anastomotic fistula. Infections occur following the invasion of pathogenic bacteria into the abdominal cavity or the involved organs. These infections mainly manifest as diffuse peritonitis, peritoneal

[*] Corresponding author: Wen-Liang Yu, MD, Department of Intensive Care Medicine, Chi Mei Medical Center, N0. 901 Chuang Hwa Road, Yung Kang District, 710 Tainan City, Taiwan. Tel.: +886-6-281-2811, ext.52605; fax: +886-6-251-7849. E-mail address: Yuleon_md@yahoo.com.tw.

abscesses, or multiple intra-abdominal visceral abscesses that require treatment combining surgical protocols with anti-infective agents. Sepsis can occur due to the invasion of numerous bacteria and toxins into the blood circulation, which may further progress to septic shock, respiratory distress syndrome, acute renal failure as well as intestinal and hepatic dysfunction.

Currently, the predominant causative bacteria include Gram-negative bacteria, such as *Escherichia coli* (*E. coli*), *Klebsiella pneumoniae (K. pneumoniae) and Pseudomonas aeruginosa (P. aeruginosa) as well as* Gram-positive bacteria like *Staphylococcus aureus* (*S. aureus*) and *Enterococcus faecalis (E. faecalis).* The widespread multi-drug resistant Gram-negative organisms are challenging physicians to effectively treat these infections.

Followed by the extensive use of broad-spectrum antibiotics, the extended-spectrum β-lactamases (ESBLs) and AmpC β-lactamases have conferred resistance of the Gram-negative organisms to third- and fourth-generation cephalosporins and have limited the choice of antibiotics to carbapenems for therapy against serious infections. As increasing use of carbapenems, however, carbapenem-resistant enterobacteria are alarmingly emerged in the field of trauma-related intra-abdominal infections. Resistance to ertapenem frequently occurs in the ESBL- and/or AmpC-producing enterobacteria with deficiency of outer membrane porin genes, such as loss or truncated mutation of *ompK35* and *ompK36* in *K. pneumoniae.* Whereas resistances to imipenem and/or meropenem usually necessity additional production of carbapenemases, such as *K. pneumoniae* carbapenemase (KPC) and New Delhi metallo-β-lactamase 1 (NDM-1).

Amikacin, gentamicin, fosfomycin, tigecycline and colistin are active versus most isolates of the KPC-producing enterobacteria, whereas only tigecycline and colistin remain active versus most NDM-1 isolates. Vancomycin and teicoplanin remain active against *S. aureus* isolates. Fosfomycin, tigecycline, daptomycin and linezolid are potential candidates to treat most Gram-positive bacteria, especially with vancomycin resistance.

In summary, surgical source control and combination therapies with the most potent anti-infective agents are indicated to treat the patients with trauma-related intra-abdominal serious infections, based on the local bacterial susceptibility epidemiology.

# INTRODUCTION

Blunt abdominal trauma can cause diffuse abdominal pain and mild to large hematoma of the anterior abdominal wall. The effect of increased pressure on colonic wall tension can lead to focal intestinal perforation, presenting with early signs of peritoneal irritation, which may not be recognized until occurrence of peritonitis, abdominal wall infection and even fulminant necrotizing fasciitis in the delayed period [1]. Necrotizing fasciitis involves widespread necrosis of the skin, subcutaneous tissue and superficial fascia, which is a potentially fatal infection and requires extensive resuscitation measures, broad-spectrum antibiotics and surgical debridement [2].

Abdominal wall trauma may develop actinomycosis, which may present as abdominal wall mass simulating a soft tissue tumor, infiltrating into the abdominal wall with adherence to the colon [3]. Actinomycosis, a chronic suppurative infection with granuloma and fibrosis, is diagnosed based on the histologic demonstration of sulfur granules in the pus or surgically resected specimen, and treatment consists of long-term penicillin-based therapies. Surgery combined with antibiotic treatment is a curative approach for this relatively rare infection.

An abdominal stabbing wound may subsequently develop an anterior abdominal wall abscess. Penetrating abdominal trauma can cause intra-abdominal infections with complications of lower lobe pneumonia related to a subphrenic abscess or of small bowel obstruction caused by an abscess compression [4]. The penetrated injury of digestive hollow organs with a small leak of colonic content may develop consecutive local peritonitis and show all signs of an acute abdomen in the early posttraumatic phase. Such injuries can lead to a profound septic shock if not appropriately treated. Abdominal gunshot injury is a life-threatening condition that requires urgent control of hemorrhage and infection through a surgical intervention or selective non-operative management, prophylaxis and antibiotic therapy of the infectious complications [5].

Initial infection process of diffuse peritonitis and bacteremia is caused by *E. coli* and *Enterococcus* spp, while the late development of abscess was caused by mixed infections with *Bacteroides fragilis* (*B. fragilis*) group and other anaerobes. The aerobic Gram-positive cocci are usually predominantly isolated from subphrenic abscess after splenectomy for abdominal trauma [6, 7]. Application of antibiotic prophylaxis or empiric antibiotic therapy should be broad-spectrum and rapidly bactericidal. This review describes the microbiology and management of intra-abdominal infections as a result of direct trauma.

## Microbial Etiology

Intra-abdominal infections following penetrating or blunt abdominal trauma often involve the gastrointestinal aerobic and anaerobic bacterial flora. The intra-abdominal infection is biphasic. The initial leakage of the endogenous gastrointestinal microflora into the peritoneal cavity results in generalized peritonitis and secondary septicemia, which is frequently followed by localized intra-abdominal abscess formation [8]. These infections are most frequently polymicrobial and are related directly to the endogenous microflora at the various levels of the gastrointestinal tract. The highest concentrations and greatest predominance of anaerobes are in the colon [9, 10]. The *Enterobacteriaceae* are the major pathogens in the peritonitis stage, and the *B. fragilis* group predominates in the abscess stage [6, 7]. The predominant aerobes and facultatives in the abdominal infections were *E. coli* and *Streptococcus* species. The predominant anaerobes were *Bacteroides*, *Peptostreptococcus* and *Clostridium* species. Of the *B. fragilis* group, *B. fragilis* accounted for 58 per cent of isolates in peritoneal aspirates and 75 per cent in aspirates from the intra-abdominal abscesses [6].

In a study for children with infections mainly after blunt trauma, the pathogens of anaerobic bacteria only (22%), aerobic bacteria only (29%), and mixed aerobic-anaerobic flora (49%) were recovered. The predominant anaerobic bacteria included *Peptostreptococcus* spp, followed by *Prevotella* spp, *Fusobacterium* spp, *B. fragilis* group, and *Clostridium* spp. The predominant aerobic bacteria were *S. aureus,* followed by *E. coli, P. aeruginosa, Streptococcus pyogenes, and K. pneumoniae* [11]. In a recent study for analyzing the bacteriology from abdominal trauma patients with severe intra-abdominal infection, the five predominant pus bacteria were *E. coli, S. aureus, K. pneumoniae, E. faecalis* and *P. aeruginosa* [12].

## Antimicrobial Resistance of the Organisms

Antimicrobial resistance among *Enterobacteriaceae* isolated from intra-abdominal infections is a global problem. A significant proportion of inducible β-lactamase (AmpC) and extended-spectrum β-lactamase (ESBL)-producing *Enterobacteriaceae* causing intra-abdominal infection were acquired in the community. In the Study for Monitoring Antimicrobial Resistance Trends (SMART) surveillance for clinical isolates from intra-abdominal infections performed in Spain from 2002 to 2010, ESBLs were detected in 8.7% of *E. coli* isolates; *K. pneumoniae*, 8.4%; *Klebsiella oxytoca*, 1.4%; and *Proteus mirabilis*, 1.6% [13]. Ertapenem and meropenem were the most active antimicrobials against ESBL producers (susceptibility, 95.5-100%) [13]. In the worldwide SMART surveillance, ESBLs were detected in 12% of *E. coli* and 18% of *Klebsiella* spp. from intra-abdominal infections in 2005 [14].

The emergence of multidrug-resistant pathogens within the clinical environment is presenting a mounting problem in hospitals worldwide. The 'ESKAPE' pathogens (*Enterococcus faecium*, *S. aureus*, *K. pneumoniae*, *Acinetobacter baumannii*, *P. aeruginosa* and *Enterobacter* spp.) [15] as well as vancomycin-resistant enterococci (VRE) have been highlighted as a group of multidrug-resistant organisms in a majority of nosocomial infections. Furthermore, emerging carbapenem resistance has been described during carbapenem therapy, leading to clinical failure [16]. Carbapenem resistance in *Enterobacteriaceae* may occur either by the acquisition of a carbapenemase, hyperproduction of AmpC or an ESBL combined with porin mutations or via efflux pumps [17].

## Perioperative Antibiotic Use

Patients sustaining penetrating abdominal injuries with colon or other hollow viscus perforation carry a high risk for postoperative infections, such as superficial surgical-site wound infections and deep surgical-site infections (fasciitis, peritonitis and intra-abdominal abscess). In a large study of 2,416 patients undergoing laparotomy for penetrating abdominal trauma, an intra-abdominal abscess developed in 2.4% patients during the postoperative period [18]. The morbidity and mortality due to wound infection, peritonitis and intra-abdominal abscess were directly proportional to the length of time from colonic injury to repair [19].

For prevention of postoperative intra-abdominal abscess in patients with penetrating abdominal trauma, preoperative antibiotic administration, careful closure of digestive tract perforation, and copious irrigation of the peritoneal cavity at the completion of surgery are necessary [18]. In a prospective double-blind trial for patients with penetrating abdominal trauma, major abdominal infections (necrotizing fasciitis, diffuse peritonitis and abscess) occurred in 8% of those receiving 1-day therapy and 10% receiving 5-day therapy with cefoxitin or cefotetan, as well as 14% with 1-day therapy and 15% with 5-day therapy, respectively, for high-risk subgroup patients with colon injury [20]. The optimal duration of preoperative antibiotic therapy is 24 hour for all penetrating abdominal trauma, regardless of peritoneal contamination and degree of colon injury [20].

In a similar prospective randomized study, perioperative antibiotic use in these high-risk patients results in surgical-site infection rates of 10% by using one preoperative and three postoperative doses of ampicillin/sulbactam 3 g intravenously for 5 days, in comparison to 8% by using the same antibiotic regimen for 1 days ($p = 0.74$). Therefore, a 24-hour course of a broad-spectrum antibiotic use can effectively prevent postoperative infections in high-risk patients sustaining hollow organ injury from penetrating abdominal trauma [21].

## ANTIMICROBIAL THERAPY

The successful treatment of intra-abdominal infection is primarily associated with prompt diagnosis and appropriate surgical intervention. Antibiotics administered parenterally are also required to decrease the incidence of local bacterial infection or septicemia [8]. The goal of antimicrobial therapy is to reduce morbidity, mortality, and duration of hospital stay. The use of antibiotic agents should have a spectrum of activity effective against the aerobic coliforms and anaerobic *B. fragilis* group [9, 10] as well as consideration of adverse drug effects and superinfection [22]. Single-agent regimens have demonstrated benefit in patients with acute intra-abdominal contamination and established infections [22]. For example in an open study, ticarcillin /clavulanate administered at a dose of 3.1 g every four or every six hours for a minimum of three days was effective in 80% of patients with intra-abdominal infections due to penetrating abdominal trauma [23]. Systemic administration of either single or in combination of newer antibiotics has been used successfully to treat intra-abdominal infection while avoiding the toxicity of aminoglycosides [24]. The primary guide for directing changes in antimicrobial therapy depends on the patient's clinical response and the culture results.

General guidelines for selecting antimicrobial agents versus intra-abdominal infections, including from patients with peritoneal contamination following abdominal trauma, are available from the Therapeutic Agents Committee of the Surgical Infection Society [25]. The applications of newer antibiotics for multidrug-resistant pathogens are reviewed here, including glycylcyclines (i.e., tigecycline), carbapenems (i.e., doripenem), oxazolidinone (i.e., linezolid, tedizolid), lipoglycopeptides (i.e., dalbavancin, telavancin, and oritavancin), and newer generation cephalosporins (i.e., ceftaroline, ceftobiprole) [26-28].

## *Enterobacteriaceae* that Express ESBL and AmpC Enzymes

ESBL-producing *Enterobacteriaceae* represent a current clinical concern as these organisms possess activity against broad-spectrum cephalosporins including third-generation (e.g., ceftriaxone, cefotaxime, ceftazidime) and fourth-generation cephalosporins (e.g., cefepime), monobactams (e.g., aztreonam), as well as novel antistaphylococcal agents such as ceftaroline [29]. During a 10 year surveillance for isolates from intra-abdominal infections in China, the ESBL rates of *E. coli* isolates increased from 36.1% in 2002-2003 to 68.1% in 2010-2011 ($p < 0.001$); whereas the ESBL rates of *K. pneumoniae* isolates remained between 30.1 and 39.3% with no significant change [30].

In addition to ESBL-type enzymes, Ambler class C (AmpC-type) enzymes may also effectively hydrolyze third-generation cephalosporins, cephamycins (e.g., cefoxitin), new anti-staphylococcal cephalosporins such as ceftaroline [29], anti-pseudomonal penicillins (such as piperacillin and ticarcillin), and their β-lactamase inhibitor combinations. High-level chromosomal AmpC enzymes are found particularly in *Enterobacter cloacae, Enterobacter aerogenes, Serratia marcescens, Citrobacter freundii, Providencia* spp., and *Morganella morganii* [31]. Plasmid-mediated AmpC is now becoming increasingly common as a cause of resistance in *K. pneumoniae* and *E. coli* [32, 33]. Furthermore, plasmid-mediated AmpC can coexist with ESBL enzymes in a single organism, making resistant profile even more complicated [32]. Cefepime is stable to AmpC-producing isolates, but efficacy against ESBL-producers is unreliable [34].

Carbapenems are generally stable to hydrolysis by ESBLs or AmpC. Carbapenems like imipenem, meropenem and doripenem have long been considered the first-line treatment option for severe infections caused by ESBL or AmpC producers [35]. Ertapenem, a carbapenem lacking activity against *Pseudomonas*, has been increasingly used for directed therapy against ESBL and AmpC producers causing mild-to-moderate infections. Tigecycline, a first in class glycylcyline, exhibits potent activity against most ESBL- and AmpC-producing *Enterobacteriaceae*, but has decreased activity against *P. aeruginosa* [36]. Ceftaroline plus amikacin appeared a promising synergistic combination against the ESBL-producing gram-negative pathogens [29]. Ceftaroline-avibactam, a novel broad-spectrum β-lactamase inhibitor combination, could be a useful therapeutic option for *Enterobacteriaceae* isolates producing ESBL or AmpC β-lactamases [37, 38].

## Carbapenem–Resistant *Enterobacteriaceae* (CRE)

Carbapenem resistance in *Enterobacteriaceae* could be attributed to production of cabapenemases alone or combination of production of ESBL or AmpC β-lactamases and deficiency of porins in the outer membrane [16, 17]. The most challenging *Enterobacteriaceae* are isolates producing KPC-type, NDM-type or oxacillinase-48 (OXA-48)-type carbapenemases, as these organisms are almost highly resistant to carbapenems and many other classes of commonly used antimicrobial agents [39]. For example, in a large collection of gram-negative pathogens from intra-abdominal infections as part of the SMART from 19 hospital sites in the United States during 2011, 41.1% of the *K. pneumoniae* (ESBL-producers) co-produced a carbapenemase (KPC-2 or KPC-3) [40].

About 26%-44% of deaths in patients with CRE infections were attributable to carbapenem resistance [41]. To date, the treatment for serious CRE infections remains difficult. In terms of in vitro susceptibility, two agents that maintain well activity against CRE are tigecycline and polymyxins (polymyxin B and colistin, so-call polymyxin E) [42]. However, in a small series of patients with bacteremia due to carbapenem-resistant *K. pneumoniae*, breakthrough bacteremia occurred in the patients all receiving tigecycline [43]. In a subgroup of *K. pneumoniae* with carbapenem resistance due to OXA-48 enzymes, the ratios of synergistic effect between fosfomycin as well as imipenem, meropenem and tigecycline were about 30% to 40%, but the combination of fosfomycin with colistin was fully antagonistic [44]. The therapeutic management of CRE may depend on the minimum inhibitory concentration (MIC) range of carbapenem (meropenem and imipenem). For *Enterobacteriaceae* with MICs of 8mg/L or less for carbapenems, a combination of carbapenem with either colistin or high-dose tigecycline (double standard dose) or aminoglycoside or even triple combinations seem to confer some therapeutic advantage over monotherapy. For *Enterobacteriaceae* with MIC higher than 8 mg/L, a combination of two or even three antibiotics among colistin, high-dose tigecycline, aminoglycoside and fosfomycin seems to confer decreased mortality [45]. Ceftaroline-avibactam is active against KPC-producing *Enterobacteriaceae* [37, 38].

## Multidrug–Resistant *P. aeruginosa*

In general, anti-pseudomonal β-lactams mainly include ceftazidime, aztreonam, cefepime, piperacillin, piperacillin/tazobactam, imipenem, meropenem and doripenem. Standard combinations against *P. aeruginosa* consist of an anti-pseudomonal β-lactam with an aminoglycoside or fluoroquinolone. Intravenous colistin-based combinations have been alternative choices to treat *P. aeruginosa* infections in the development of multiple resistances to anti-pseudomonal β-lactams [46-48].

## Carbapenem–Resistant *A. baumannii* (CRAB)

Carbapenems have generally been considered the agents of choice for treatment of infections caused by *A. baumannii*, owing to their intrinsic activity against this organism. However, *A. baumannii* has emerged as a potent nosocomial pathogen with resistance to broad-spectrum β-lactams, aminoglycosides, fluoroquinolones, and most notably, carbapenems. The most significant mechanism of carbapenem resistance in *A. baumannii* is the production of OXA-group carbapenemases (such as OXA-23, -40, -51, -58, -143, and -235) and recently, NDM-1 [49-52].

CRAB usually remains susceptible to sulbactam, polymyxins (colistin or polymyxin B) and tigecycline. Sulbactam is a β-lactamase inhibitor and also has affinity for penicillin-binding proteins of *A. baumannii* [53]. In a study of treating invasive CRAB infections from Brazil, ampicillin-sulbactam with a median daily dose of 9g corresponded to a 60% clinical response rate [54].

Colistin is the more commonly used polymyxin formulation worldwide, and clinical experience showed that polymyxin resistance can develop after treatment with colistin, especially when patients are exposed to suboptimal concentrations of colistin [55]. Therefore, the use of a loading dose (6-MU) and combination therapy is now advocated for colistin therapy [56-58]. The synergistic ratios of colistin with imipenem and sulbactam were 88% and 92%, respectively [58].

Tigecycline is a semisynthetic derivative of minocycline that has a broader spectrum of activity against multi-drug resistant organisms, including *A. baumannii*. However, resistance to tigecycline in *A. baumannii* may develop through overexpression of efflux pumps [59, 60]. Therefore, tigecycline monotherapy is not recommended for multidrug-resistant *A. baumannii* infection, but tigecycline combined with colistin or cephoperazone/ sulbactam seemed to yield a good clinical outcome for multidrug-resistant *A. baumannii* infection [61]. The combinations of tigecycline with sulbactam or rifampin also showed good in vitro activities against multidrug-resistant *A. baumannii* isolates [62].

## Methicillin-Resistant *Staphylococcus aureus* (MRSA)

In the treatment of MRSA, glycopeptides (vancomycin and teicoplanin) remain drugs of choice. Daptomycin is currently the only antibiotic to have shown not inferiority to vancomycin in the treatment of MRSA bacteremia and right-sided endocarditis [63]. Refractory MRSA peritonitis was ever successfully treated by intra-peritoneal daptomycin combined with oral rifampin in a patient receiving peritoneal dialysis [64]. Linezolid should be considered an option in the treatment for patients with proven MRSA pneumonia [65]. However, a patient with peritoneal dialysis-related peritonitis caused by MRSA developed linezolid-resistant MRSA while being treated with linezolid [66]. Tedizolid, a novel oxazolidinone, is more potent but with less adverse effects than its comparator linezolid [67, 68]. Tedizolid is recently approved for the treatment of acute bacterial skin and skin structure infections caused by susceptible Gram-positive pathogens, including MRSA. Importantly, tedizolid demonstrates activity against linezolid-resistant bacterial strains [68].

Tigecycline received approval by the United States Food and Drug Administration (FDA) for treatment of complicated skin and skin structure and intra abdominal infections [26]. Tigecycline has in vitro activity against many gram-positive bacteria and achieves high clinical success rates of more than 90% in patients with documented intra-abdominal infections caused by multidrug-resistant bacteria, including MRSA [69].

Lipoglycopeptides (dalbavancin, telavancin, and oritavancin) show in vitro potency and pharmacodynamics properties greater than vancomycin [67,

70, 71]. Anti-MRSA cephalosporins (ceftobiprole and ceftaroline) with high affinity for the penicillin-binding protein PBP2a offer great promise in the treatment of MRSA infections, including acute bacterial skin and skin structure infections and pneumonia [67, 71-73]. Currently, there are no published data for the treatment of MRSA intra-abdominal infections with lipoglycopeptides and anti-MRSA cephalosporins.

### Vancomycin-Resistant *Enterococcus* (VRE)

Concerning the widespread use of vancomycin, the prevalence of VRE has risen rapidly in many countries and has become a significant problem in terms of nosocomial infection [74]. Few reports have been published for successful treatment using new agents with activity against VRE - such as linezolid and daptomycin for peritoneal dialysis -associated VRE peritonitis [75, 76]. Linezolid, which has bacteriostatic activity, is approved for the treatment of VRE infections and bacteremia by the United States FDA. Meanwhile, daptomycin exerts bactericidal activity against VRE, but is not approved for the treatment of VRE bacteremia. A recent meta-analysis of 13 studies shows that linezolid treatment for VRE bacteremia was associated with a lower mortality than daptomycin treatment [77]. Linezolid provided high rates of clinical cure and microbiological success in VRE and MRSA complicated infections, including intra-abdominal infections [78]. Tedizolid is four- to eightfold more potent in vivo than linezolid against all species of staphylococci, enterococci, and streptococci, including MRSA and VRE [68]. Tigecycline achieved high clinical success rates in patients with documented infections involving multi-resistant bacteria strains, including intra-abdominal infections caused by VRE [69].

## Conclusion

The abdominal trauma includes blunt trauma, lacerations and penetration injuries. Principal infections associated with trauma were wounds, fasciitis, peritonitis, bacteremia, and abscesses. An urgent surgical intervention is the mainstay of the management of serious intra-abdominal infections. Simple abscesses may be percutaneously drained; while complex abscesses often require open surgical drainage. Abdominal trauma – associated intra-abdominal infections often involve the gastrointestinal aerobic and anaerobic bacterial flora. The intra-abdominal infection is biphasic, with the *Enterobacteriaceae* as the major pathogens in the peritonitis stage, and the *B. fragilis* group predominant in the abscess stage. Among isolates from abdominal abscesses, anaerobic bacteria alone were present in about 15-20%, aerobes alone in 2-20%%, and mixed flora in 50-80%. Single or combined antimicrobial agent is mandatory for effective therapy against both *Enterobacteriaceae* and the *B. fragilis* group. The optimal duration of preoperative antibiotic therapy is 24 hour for all penetrating abdominal trauma, regardless of degree of colon injury and peritoneal contamination. Some second-generation and third-generation cephalosporins are often efficient, cost-effective and safe in treating intra-abdominal infections. The carbapenems are considered appropriate for the treatment of severe intra-abdominal infections caused by ESBL- or AmpC producers. The treatment of CRE-associated infections usually requires a combination of two or three agents of carbapenem, colistin, tigecycline, fosfomycin and/or aminoglycoside. Vancomycin and teicoplanin remain active against *S. aureus*. Fosfomycin, tigecycline, daptomycin, linezolid, tedizolid, lipoglycopeptides and anti-MRSA cephalosporins are potential candidates to treat most Gram-positive bacteria, especially with vancomycin resistance.

## References

[1] Pecic, V; Nestorovic, M; Kovacevic, P; Tasic, D; Stanojevic, G. Catastrophic necrotizing fasciitis after blunt abdominal trauma with delayed recognition of the coecal rupture - case report. *Ulus. Travma Acil. Cerrahi. Derg.*, 2014, 20, 143-146.

[2] Martínez-Pérez, A; Garrigós-Ortega, G; Gómez-Abril, SÁ; Martí-Martínez, E; Torres-Sánchez, T. Traumatic abdominal hernia complicated by necrotizing fasciitis. *Ulus. Travma. Acil. Cerrahi. Derg.*, 2014, 20, 455-458.

[3] Ozcan, R; Mammadov, E; Aydin, E; Adaletli, I; Esen, T; Dervisoglu, S; et al. Actinomycosis presenting as an abdominal mass in a child. *APSP J. Case Rep.*, 2011, 2, 4.

[4] Singh, S; Khardori, NM. Intra-abdominal and pelvic emergencies. *Med. Clin. North. Am.*, 2012, 96, 1171-1191.

[5] Lamb, CM; Garner, JP. Selective non-operative management of civilian gunshot wounds to the abdomen, a systematic review of the evidence. *Injury*, 2014, 45, 659-666.

[6] Brook, I. A 12 year study of aerobic and anaerobic bacteria in intra-abdominal and postsurgical abdominal wound infections. *Surg. Gynecol. Obstet.*, 1989, 169, 387-392.

[7] Brook, I. Management of infection following intra-abdominal trauma. *Ann. Emerg. Med.*, 1988, 17, 626-632.

[8] Nichols, RL. Management of intra-abdominal sepsis. *Am. J. Med.*, 1986, 80, 204-209.

[9] Nichols, RL. Intra-abdominal sepsis, controversies and choices in management. *Clin. Ther.,* 1987, 10, S50-58.

[10] Nichols, RL. The treatment of intraabdominal infections in surgery. *Diagn. Microbiol. Infect. Dis.*, 1989, 12, S195-199.

[11] Brook, I. Aerobic and anaerobic microbiology of infections after trauma in children. *J. Accid. Emerg. Med.*, 1998, 15, 162-167.

[12] Zhang, S; Ren, L; Li, Y; Wang, J; Yu, W; Li, N; Li, J. Bacteriology and drug susceptibility analysis of pus from patients with severe intra-abdominal infection induced by abdominal trauma. *Exp. Ther. Med.*, 2014, 7, 1427-1431.

[13] Cantón, R; Loza, E; Aznar, J; Calvo, J; Cercenado, E; Cisterna, R, et al, SMART-Spain Working Group. Antimicrobial susceptibility of Gram-negative organisms from intraabdominal infections and evolution of isolates with extended spectrum β-lactamases in the SMART study in Spain (2002-2010). *Rev. Esp. Quimioter.*, 2011, 24, 223-232.

[14] Baquero, F; Hsueh, PR; Paterson, DL; Rossi, F; Bochicchio, GV; Gallagher, G, et al. In vitro susceptibilities of aerobic and facultatively anaerobic gram-negative bacilli isolated from patients with intra-abdominal infections worldwide, 2005 results from Study for Monitoring Antimicrobial Resistance Trends (SMART). *Surg. Infect. (Larchmt)*, 2009, 10, 99-104.

[15] Boucher, HW; Talbot, GH; Bradley, JS; Edwards, JE; Gilbert, D; Rice, LB; et al. Bad bugs, no drugs, no ESKAPE! An update from the Infectious Diseases Society of America. *Clin. Infect. Dis.*, 2009, 48, 1-12.

[16] Skurnik, D; Lasocki, S; Bremont, S; Muller-Serieys, C; Kitzis, MD; Courvalin, P; et al. Development of ertapenem resistance in a patient with mediastinitis caused by *Klebsiella pneumoniae* producing an extended-spectrum β-lactamase. *J. Med. Microbiol.,* 2010, 59, 115–119.

[17] Suh, B; Bae, IK; Kim, J; Jeong, SH; Yong, D; Lee, K. Outbreak of meropenem-resistant *Serratia marcescens* comediated by chromosomal

AmpC β-lactamase overproduction and outer membrane protein loss. *Antimicrob. Agents Chemother.,* 2010, 54, 5057–5061.

[18] Gibson, DM; Feliciano, DV; Mattox, KL; Gentry, LO; Jordan, GL. Jr. Intraabdominal abscess after penetrating abdominal trauma. *Am. J. Surg.*, 1981, 142, 699-703.

[19] Matolo, NM; Cohen, SE; Wolfman, EF. Jr. Experimental evaluation of primary repair of colonic injuries. *Arch. Surg.*, 1976, 111, 78-80.

[20] Fabian, TC; Croce, MA; Payne, LW; Minard, G; Pritchard, FE; Kudsk, KA. Duration of antibiotic therapy for penetrating abdominal trauma, a prospective trial. *Surgery*, 1992, 112, 788-794, discussion 794-795.

[21] Kirton, OC; O'Neill, PA; Kestner, M; Tortella, BJ. Perioperative antibiotic use in high-risk penetrating hollow viscus injury, a prospective randomized, double-blind, placebo-control trial of 24 hours versus 5 days. *J. Trauma*, 2000, 49, 822-832.

[22] DiPiro, JT. Considerations for therapy of mixed infections, focus on intraabdominal infection. *Pharmacotherapy*, 1995, 15, S15-21.

[23] Levine, DP; Wilson, RF. Treatment of penetrating abdominal trauma and gynecologic infections. *J. Reprod. Med.*, 1988, 33, S598-602.

[24] Malangoni, MA. Pathogenesis and treatment of intra-abdominal infection. *Surg. Gynecol. Obstet.*, 1990, 171, S31-S34.

[25] Mazuski, JE; Sawyer, RG; Nathens, AB; DiPiro, JT; Schein, M; Kudsk, KA; et al., Therapeutic Agents Committee of the Surgical Infections Society. The Surgical Infection Society guidelines on antimicrobial therapy for intra-abdominal infections, evidence for the recommendations. *Surg. Infect. (Larchmt),* 2002, 3, 175-233.

[26] Bosso, JA. The antimicrobial armamentarium, evaluating current and future treatment options. *Pharmacotherapy*, 2005, 25, S55-62.

[27] Weber, DJ; Rutala, WA. New antibiotic agents, problems and prospects. *Surg. Infect. (Larchmt)*, 2005, 6, S-97-107.

[28] Hasper, D; Schefold, JC; Baumgart, DC. Management of severe abdominal infections. *Recent Pat. Antiinfect. Drug Discov.*, 2009, 4, 57-65.

[29] Vidaillac, C; Leonard, SN; Sader, HS; Jones, RN; Rybak, MJ. In vitro activity of ceftaroline alone and in combination against clinical isolates of resistant gram-negative pathogens, including β-lactamase-producing *Enterobacteriaceae* and *Pseudomonas aeruginosa. Antimicrob. Agents Chemother.*, 2009, 53, 2360-2366.

[30] Yang, Q; Zhang, H; Wang, Y; Xu, Y; Chen, M; Badal, RE; et al. A 10 year surveillance for antimicrobial susceptibility of *Escherichia coli* and

*Klebsiella pneumoniae* in community- and hospital-associated intra-abdominal infections in China. *J. Med. Microbiol.,* 2013, 62, 1343-1349.

[31] Jones, RN. Important and emerging β-lactamase-mediated resistances in hospital-based pathogens, the Amp C enzymes. *Diagn. Microbiol. Infect. Dis.*, 1998, 31, 461-466.

[32] Alvarez, M; Tran, JH; Chow, N; Jacoby, GA. Epidemiology of conjugative plasmid-mediated AmpC β-lactamases in the United States. *Antimicrob. Agents Chemother.*, 2004, 48, 533–537.

[33] Reuland, EA; Hays, JP; de, Jongh, DM; Abdelrehim, E; Willemsen, I; Kluytmans, JA; et al. Detection and occurrenceof plasmid-mediated AmpC in highly resistant gram-negativerods. *PLoS. ONE*, 2014, 9, e91396.

[34] Harris, PN. Clinical management of infections caused by *Enterobacteriaceae* that express extended-spectrum β-lactamase and AmpC enzymes. *Semin. Respir. Crit. Care Med.*, 2015, 36, 56-73.

[35] Pfaller, MA; Jones, RN. MYSTIC (Meropenem Yearly Susceptibility Test Information Collection) results from the Americas, resistance implications in the treatment of serious infections. *J. Antimicrob. Chemother.,* 2000, 46, S25-37.

[36] Sader, HS; Jones, RN; Dowzicky, MJ; Fritsche, TR. Antimicrobial activity of tigecycline tested against nosocomial bacterial pathogens from patients hospitalized in the intensive care unit. *Diagn. Microbiol. Infect. Dis.*, 2005, 52, 203-208.

[37] Castanheira, M; Williams, G; Jones, RN; Sader, HS. Activity of ceftaroline-avibactam tested against contemporary Enterobacteriaceae isolates carrying β-lactamases prevalent in the United States. *Microb. Drug Resist.*, 2014, 20, 436-440.

[38] Li, H; Estabrook, M; Jacoby, GA; Nichols, WW; Testa, RT; Bush, K. In vitro susceptibility of characterized β-lactamase-producing strains tested with avibactam combinations. *Antimicrob. Agents Chemother.*, 2015, 59, 1789-1793.

[39] Nordmann, P. Carbapenemase-producing *Enterobacteriacea*e, overview of a major public health challenge. *Med. Mal. Infect.*, 2014, 44, 51-56.

[40] Hawser, SP; Badal, RE; Bouchillon, SK; Hoban, DJ; Hackel, MA; Biedenbach, DJ; et al. Susceptibility of gram-negative aerobic bacilli from intra-abdominal pathogens to antimicrobial agents collected in the United States during 2011. *J. Infect.*, 2014, 68, 71-76.

[41] Falagas, ME; Tansarli, GS; Karageorgopoulos, DE; Vardakas, KZ. Deaths attributable to carbapenem-resistant *Enterobacteriaceae* infections. *Emerg. Infect. Dis.*, 2014, 20, 1170-1175.

[42] Perez, F; Van, Duin, D. Carbapenem-resistant *Enterobacteriaceae*, a menace to our most vulnerable patients. *Cleve. Clin. J. Med.*, 2013, 80, 225-233.

[43] Nguyen, M; Eschenauer, GA; Bryan, M; O'Neil, K; Furuya, EY; Della-Latta, P; et al. Carbapenem-resistant *Klebsiella pneumoniae* bacteremia, factors correlated with clinical and microbiologic outcomes. *Diagn. Microbiol. Infect. Dis.*, 2010, 67, 180-184.

[44] Evren, E; Azap, OK; Çolakoğlu, Ş; Arslan, H. In vitro activity of fosfomycin in combination with imipenem, meropenem, colistin and tigecycline against OXA 48-positive *Klebsiella pneumoniae* strains. *Diagn. Microbiol. Infect. Dis.*, 2013, 76, 335-338.

[45] Rafailidis, PI; Falagas, ME. Options for treating carbapenem-resistant *Enterobacteriaceae. Curr. Opin. Infect. Dis.*, 2014, 27, 479-483.

[46] Tascini, C; Gemignani, G; Ferranti, S; Tagliaferri, E; Leonildi, A; Lucarini, A; et al. Microbiological activity and clinical efficacy of a colistin and rifampin combination in multidrug-resistant *Pseudomonas aeruginosa* infections. *J. Chemother.,* 2004, 16, 282-287.

[47] D'Souza, BB; Padmaraj, SR; Rekha, PD; Tellis, RC; Prabhu, S; Pothen, P. In vitro synergistic activity of colistin and ceftazidime or ciprofloxacin against multidrug-resistant clinical strains of *Pseudomonas aeruginosa. Microb. Drug Resist.*, 2014, 20, 550-554.

[48] Lora-Tamayo, J; Murillo, O; Bergen, PJ; Nation, RL; Poudyal, A; Luo, X; et al. Activity of colistin combined with doripenem at clinically relevant concentrations against multidrug-resistant *Pseudomonas aeruginosa* in an in vitro dynamic biofilm model. *J. Antimicrob. Chemother., 2014,* 69, 2434-2442.

[49] Mugnier, PD; Poirel, L; Naas, T; Nordmann, P. Worldwide disseminationof the blaOXA-23 carbapenemase gene of *Acinetobacter baumannii. Emerg. Infect. Dis.*, 2010, 16, 35–40.

[50] Chen, Y; Zhou, Z; Jiang, Y; Yu, Y. Emergence of NDM-1-producing *Acinetobacter baumannii* in China. *J. Antimicrob. Chemother.,* 2011, 66, 1255–1259.

[51] Higgins, PG; Pérez-Llarena, FJ; Zander, E; Fernández, A; Bou, G; Seifert, H. OXA-235, a novel class D β-lactamase involved in resistance to carbapenems in *Acinetobacter baumannii. Antimicrob. Agents Chemother.,* 2013, 57, 2121–2126.

[52] Decousser, JW; Jansen, C; Nordmann, P; Emirian, A; Bonnin, RA; Anais, L; et al. Outbreak of NDM-1-producing *Acinetobacter baumannii* in France, January to May 2013. *Euro. Surveill.,* 2013, 18, 20547.
[53] Noguchi, JK; Gill, MA. Sulbactam, a β-lactamase inhibitor. *Clin. Pharm.,* 1988, 7, 37–51.
[54] Oliveira, MS; Prado, GV; Costa, SF; Grinbaum, RS; Levin, AS. Ampicillin/sulbactam compared with polymyxins for the treatment of infections caused by carbapenem-resistant *Acinetobacter* spp. *J. Antimicrob. Chemother.,* 2008, 61, 1369–1375.
[55] Qureshi, ZA; Hittle, LE; O'Hara, JA; Rivera, JI; Syed, A; Shields, RK; et al. Colistin-resistant *Acinetobacter baumannii,* beyond carbapenem resistance. *Clin. Infect. Dis.*, 2015, 60, 1295-1303.
[56] MohamedAF; Karaiskos, I; PlachourasD; Karvanen, M; Pontikis, K; Jansson, B; et al. Application of a loading dose of colistin methane sulfonate in critically ill patients, population pharmacokinetics, protein binding, and prediction of bacterial kill. Antimicrob. *Agents Chemother.,* 2012, 56, 4241–4249.
[57] Garnacho-Montero, J; Amaya-Villar, R; Ferrándiz-Millón, C; Díaz-Martín, A; López-Sánchez, JM. Gutiérrez-Pizarraya A. Optimum treatment strategies for carbapenem-resistant *Acinetobacter baumannii* bacteremia. *Expert Rev. Anti. Infect. Ther.,* 2015, 13, 769-777.
[58] Wei, W; Yang, H; Liu, Y; Ye, Y; Li, J. In vitro synergy of colistin combinations against extensively drug-resistant *Acinetobacter baumannii* producing OXA-23 carbapenemase. *J. Chemother.,* 2015 May 15, 1973947815Y0000000030.
[59] Peleg, AY; Potoski, BA; Rea, R; Adams, J; Sethi, J; Capitano, B; et al. *Acinetobacter baumannii* blood stream infection while receiving tigecycline, a cautionary report. *J. Antimicrob. Chemother.,* 2007, 59, 128–131.
[60] Ruzin, A; Keeney, D; Bradford, PA. AdeABC multidrug efflux pump is associated with decreased susceptibility to tigecycline in *Acinetobacter calcoaceticus-Acinetobacter baumannii* complex. *J. Antimicrob. Chemother.*, 2007, 59, 1001–1004.
[61] Wu, MT; Chen, HY; Ou, TY; Kuo, LN; Cheng, KJ; Lee, WS. Clinical evaluation of tigecycline in the treatment of nosocomial infection in a hospital in Taiwan. *Int. J. Clin. Pharmacol. Ther.,* 2014, 52, 1030-1036.
[62] Dong, X; Chen, F; Zhang, Y; Liu, H; Liu, Y; Ma, L. In vitro activities of rifampin, colistin, sulbactam and tigecycline tested alone and in

combination against extensively drug-resistant *Acinetobacter baumannii. J. Antibiot. (Tokyo),* 2014, 67, 677-680.

[63] Fowler, VG, Jr; Boucher, HW; Corey, GR; Abrutyn, E; Karchmer, AW; Rupp, ME; et al. *S. aureus* Endocarditisand Bacteremia Study Group. Daptomycin versus standard therapyfor bacteremia and endocarditis caused by *Staphylococcus aureus. N. Engl. J. Med.*, 2006, 355, 653–665.

[64] Lin, SY; Ho, MW; Liu, JH; Liu, YL; Yeh, HC; Hsieh, TL; et al. Successful salvage of peritoneal catheter in unresolved methicillin-resistant *Staphylococcus aureus* peritonitis by combination treatment with daptomycin and rifampin. *Blood Purif.*, 2011, 32, 249-252.

[65] Rodvold, KA; McConeghy, KW. Methicillin-resistant *Staphylococcus aureus* therapy, past, present, and future. *Clin. Infect. Dis.*, 2014, 58, S20-7.

[66] Tsiodras, S; Gold, HS; Sakoulas, G; Eliopoulis, GM; Wennersten, C; Venkataraman, L; et al. Linezolid resistance in a clinical isolate of *Staphylococcus aureus*. *Lancet*, 2001, 358, 207–208.

[67] Holmes, NE; Howden, BP. What's new in the treatment of serious MRSA infection? *Curr. Opin. Infect. Dis.*, 2014, 27, 471-478.

[68] Zhanel, GG; Love, R; Adam, H; Golden, A; Zelenitsky, S; Schweizer, F; et al. Tedizolid, a novel oxazolidinone with potent activity against multidrug-resistant gram-positive pathogens. *Drugs*, 2015, 75, 253-270.

[69] Heizmann, WR; Löschmann, PA; Eckmann, C; von, Eiff, C; Bodmann, KF; Petrik, C. Clinical efficacy of tigecycline used as monotherapy or in combination regimens for complicated infections with documented involvement of multiresistant bacteria. *Infection,* 2015, 43, 37-43.

[70] Manfredi, R; Sabbatani, S. Novel pharmaceutical molecules against emerging resistant gram-positive cocci. *Braz. J. Infect. Dis.*, 2010, 14, 96-108.

[71] Holmes, NE; Tong, SY; Davis, JS; Hal, SJ. Treatment of methicillin-resistant *Staphylococcus aureus*, vancomycin and beyond. *Semin. Respir. Crit. Care Med.*, 2015, 36, 17-30.

[72] Chambers, HF. Ceftobiprole, in-vivo profile of a bactericidal cephalosporin. *Clin. Microbiol. Infect.,* 2006, 12, S17–S22.

[73] Steed, ME; Rybak, MJ. Ceftaroline, a new cephalosporin withactivity against resistant gram-positive pathogens. *Pharmacotherapy*, 2010, 30, 375–389.

[74] McGeer, AJ; Low, DE. Vancomycin-resistant enterococci. *Semin. Respir. Infect.*, 2000, 15, 314-326.

[75] Huen, SC; Hall, I; Topal, J; Mahnensmith, RL; Brewster, UC; Abu-Alfa, AK. Successful use of intraperitoneal daptomycin in the treatment of vancomycin-resistant *Enterococcus* peritonitis. *Am. J. Kidney Dis.*, 2009, 54, 538–541.

[76] Song, IJ; Seo, JW; Kwon, YE; Kim, YL; Lim, TS; Kang, EW; et al. Successful treatment of vancomycin-resistant enterococcus peritonitis using linezolid without catheter removal in a peritoneal dialysis patient. *Perit. Dial. Int.*, 2014, 34, 235-239.

[77] Chuang, YC; Wang, JT; Lin, HY; Chang, SC. Daptomyc in versus linezolid for treatment of vancomycin-resistant enterococcal bacteremia, systematic review and meta-analysis. *BMC. Infect. Dis.*, 2014, 14, 687. doi, 10.1186/s12879-014-0687-9.

[78] Birmingham, MC; Rayner, CR; Meagher, AK; Flavin, SM; Batts, DH; Schentag, JJ. Linezolid for the treatment of multidrug-resistant, gram-positive infections, experience from a compassionate-use program. *Clin. Infect. Dis.*, 2003, 36, 159-168.

In: Abdominal Trauma ...
Editor: Louise Santiago

ISBN: 978-1-63483-482-7


*Chapter 4*

# SERIOUS ABDOMINAL CONSEQUENCES OF FALLS AND NON-PENETRATING 'MINOR' ABDOMINAL TRAUMA AMONG OLDER ADULTS

***Ami Schattner*, MD, Eli Mavor, MD and Meital Adi, MD***

Departments of Medicine (AS), Surgery (EM) and Radiology (AM), Kaplan Medical Center, Rehovot;
Hebrew University and Hadassah Medical School, Jerusalem, Israel

## ABSTRACT

Elderly community-dwelling patients often experience ground-level falls: one out of three adults aged 65 and older falls each year and the incidence increases to 50% in those over 80 years old. Following a fall, the patient is usually brought to the emergency department where fractures or brain injury are the major concern and serious abdominal injury is seldom contemplated.

We used a retrospective chart analysis to identify all such patients presenting after a simple fall and admitted with serious blunt abdominal trauma to a single academic medical centre. Out of 546 patients screened, 3 cases of ground-level falls leading to splenic rupture; isolated

* Correspondence: Ami Schattner, MD, Professor of Medicine, Hebrew University and Hadassah Medical School, Jerusalem, Israel, Phone 972 8 939 0330, Fax 972 8 9441 187, e-mail amischatt@gmail.com

gallbladder rupture with gallstone ileus; and perinephric hematoma were found (0.55%) and are reported. The literature on other serious abdominal consequences of falls and non-penetrating 'minor' abdominal trauma among older adults not encountered in our series was reviewed to capture the whole spectrum of abdominal adverse events of falls in elderly patients. In conclusion, Falls in elderly patients are exceedingly common mandating recognition of even rare complications. Physicians should be more aware of the possibility of occult and serious consequences of blunt abdominal trauma after falls among older adults, albeit rare.

## INTRODUCTION

Falls in older persons are a common and serious problem. One out of three adults aged 65 and older falls each year [1, 2] and the incidence increases to 50% in those over 80 years old. One fall, which may not even come to the attention of the patient's provider, is the harbinger of recurrences - over half of those with a history of a fall in the previous year will have a subsequent fall [3]. Falls usually occur in elderly patients with impairments in multiple domains [2] and often have profound consequences. One prospective study of falls among 325 community dwelling individuals revealed that 55% of falls resulted in soft tissue injury and 6% were associated with a major injury such as fractures, dislocations or a laceration requiring suture [3]. Moreover, one in four falls caused the patient to limit his or her activities and many patients are left with much uncertainty and insecurity affecting their daily life and quality of life. A prospective population-based study in Finland showed that among the independent elderly, the risk of a fall resulting in major injury was high among the subjects who had peripheral neuropathy (odds ratio = 2.5) or were suffering from insomnia (odds ratio = 4.1) [4]. Thus, side by side with superficial lacerations and hematomas - hip, vertebral and other bone fractures as well as traumatic brain injury (TBI) are important causes of prolonged morbidity, dependence and early mortality in this age group [5-7]. For example, population-based surveillance data from Florida reveal that a large proportion of falls among older persons were associated with injury events and resulted in hospital admission with a mean length of stay of 11.2 days [5]. About 50% of these patients were discharged to a nursing home.

However, unrecognized by many clinicians [8], falls may also be a cause of blunt abdominal trauma which may be clinically-unapparent, present a considerable diagnostic challenge and cause diagnostic delay [9]. We decided to study this problem systematically, after encountering one such patient whose presentation and course were very unusual (Case 2). A retrospective chart review identified altogether 3 independent, community-dwelling elderly patients who fell and sustained severe abdominal trauma. This series and literature review serves to heighten primary care physicians' and emergency physicians' awareness of occult rupture or contusion of intra-abdominal organs – a rare, life-threatening complication of falls in older, community-dwelling adults.

## RISK FACTORS

Normally, homeostatic mechanisms act to maintain postural stability and prevent falls. In older persons, disruption of these mechanisms often combines with multiple morbidities, polypharmacy and obtundation of sensory input (vision, proprioception, etc.) and reduced muscle mass and function to impair balance and facilitate falls. Such disruption is very common and may be associated with any acute illness, intake of a new drug, a change to unfamiliar surroundings or slippery walking surface. Usually, there are multiple risk factors at work in the elderly patient and falls are almost never due to a single cause. The most commonly identified risk factors for repeated falls reported in most studies include older age, leg weakness or state after cerebrovascular accident, orthostatic hypotension and/or dizziness, balance problems, cognitive impairment, use of psychotropic drugs and joint pain in the legs or leg weakness. In one well known study of community dwelling elderly persons for example, the adjusted odds ratio for sedative use was 28; for cognitive impairment 5.0; and for disability of the lower extremities almost 4.0 (9). The risk of falling increased linearly with the number of risk factors (9, 10). In addition a history of a fall in the past was found to be a strong predictor of future falls [11, 12]. Interestingly, a number of simple clinical tests were found to be predictive of falls:

- Dizziness upon standing
- Orthostatic hypotension
- Standing systolic blood pressure < 110 mm Hg
- Difficulty and slowing in standing from a chair
- Having trouble bending down
- Limitations in basic activities of daily living (ADL)

Many of these clinical tests are also efficiently covered by the tested "get up and go" test, although later meta-analysis questioned its predictive value in independent older adults [13].

- Failure to perform the "functional reach" test [14].

More recently, an important study of over 3000 community-dwelling men aged 67 years or more focused on sleep disturbances as a risk factors for falls. Both subjective reports (e.g., excessive daytime sleepiness, total sleep time, etc.) and objective findings (e.g., sleep-associated breathing disturbances) were found to be significantly associated with increased risk of recurrent falls [15].

## Methods

Computer-based retrospective chart review was undertaken in an academic general hospital. All patients aged 65 or more, presenting with a fall occurring in the community and admitted to the departments of Medicine, Geriatrics, Surgery or Urology over one year (1.1 to 31.12.2012) were included if the admission diagnoses included rupture or significant trauma of an internal (abdominal) organ [16]. In addition, we reviewed the literature (PubMed, abstracted articles, English language, since inception) to identify additional types of serious internal trauma following 'simple' ground-level falls or other non-penetrating ‘minor’ abdominal trauma in elderly patients and evaluate data on their prevalence.

## Results

Altogether, 3 patients were identified out of 546 admitted patients meeting our inclusion criteria (0.55%) [16] and are reported in detail.

### Case 1

A 70-year-old woman presented to the emergency department from her home after a fall. She had a history of hypertension, obesity and depression with recent (one year) cognitive decline and occasional falls. The fall occurred after she got up at night to urinate. On her way back to bed she became dizzy and fell on her back with a brief syncope associated with fecal incontinence, vomiting (once) and cold sweat.

In the emergency department no bruising was found. Her blood pressure was 80/45 but this soon normalized with intravenous saline infusion (118/70) and her other vital signs, examination, ECG, chest X-ray and head CT were normal. She was admitted to the department of medicine and treated with ceftriaxone for fever and pyuria, intermittently complaining of pain in her back below the Lt. scapula.

On the $4^{th}$ hospital day a marked tenderness was noted over that area, and the hemoglobin gradually dropped from 12 g/dL on admission to 7.7 g/dL with systolic blood pressure of 108 mmHg, tachycardia (104/min) and pre-renal azotemia all suggesting a hypovolemic shock. CT revealed rupture of the spleen with bleeding, fractures in the lower left ribs and a small left pleural effusion (Figure 1).

Immediate surgery confirmed stage 4 rupture of the spleen and total splenectomy was done with suction of 2 liters of blood from the abdominal cavity. The patient was followed up uneventfully for over a year.

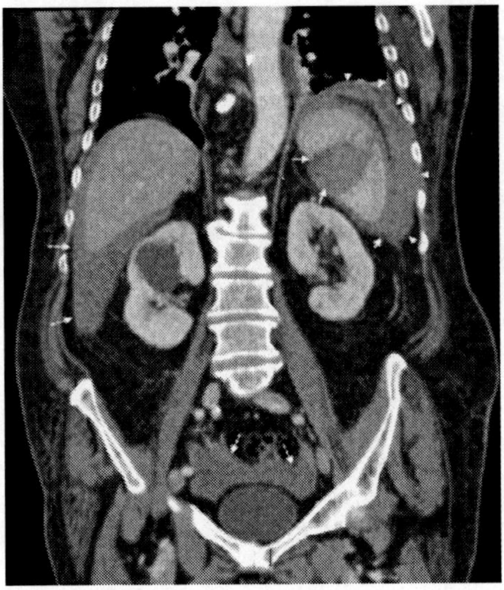

Figure 1. Contrast enhanced abdominal CT in coronal view showing splenic lacerations (solid arrows), peri-splenic hematoma (arrowheads) and hemoperitoneum (dashed arrows).

## Case 2

An independent 86-year-old woman was admitted to surgery from the emergency department 4 days after she fell at home. She had a history of diabetes, hypertension, anemia and a single hospital admission for acute cholecystitis four years prior which was treated conservatively. Cholecystectomy was then refused. After her fall, she developed gradually increasing abdominal pain associated with recurrent vomiting, diarrhea and dyspnea.

At the emergency department her vital signs were normal but her abdomen was distended and tender and a right-sided hematoma was noted.

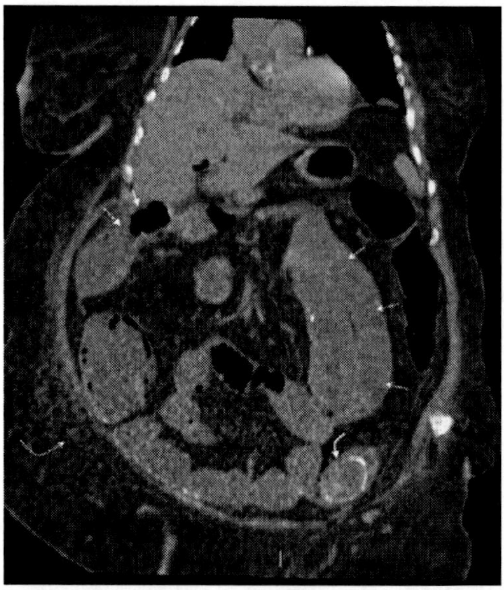

Figure 2. Coronal non-enhanced abdominal CT showing air inside the gallbladder (short solid arrow) and intra-hepatic bile ducts (long solid arrow); a fistula between the gallbladder and the hepatic flexure of the colon (dashed arrow) and a large gallstone in the distal descending colon (curved solid arrow). Dilated small bowel loops ( short dotted arrows), pneumatosis in the cecal wall (long dotted arrows) and subcutaneus hematoma in the right abdominal wall (curved dotted arrow) can also be seen.

Abdominal X-ray showed small bowel obstruction. CT demonstrated air-fluid level within a gallbladder adherent to the colon at the hepatic flexure. A large gallstone was lodged in the distal descending colon obstructing the colon which was dilated with pneumatosis intestinalis (Figure 2). Diagnosed as gallstone ileus the patient was urgently operated on. A fistula was identified between the colon and gallbladder. An ischemic-looking small and large bowel mandated cholecystectomy, total colectomy and partial resection of small bowel creating an ileostomy. The patient was then successfully treated for septic shock and multi-organ failure but remained ventilated and died four months later.

## Case 3

An independent 82-year-old man fell in the street and was injured in his left loin. He was brought to the emergency department after he had macroscopic hematuria at home. His past medical history included hypertension, cerebrovascular accident (CVA) , moderate aortic stenosis, right nephrectomy for hypernephroma eight years prior without evidence of recurrence and chronic renal failure (creatinine 2.5 mg/dL). He was not on anticoagulant treatment.

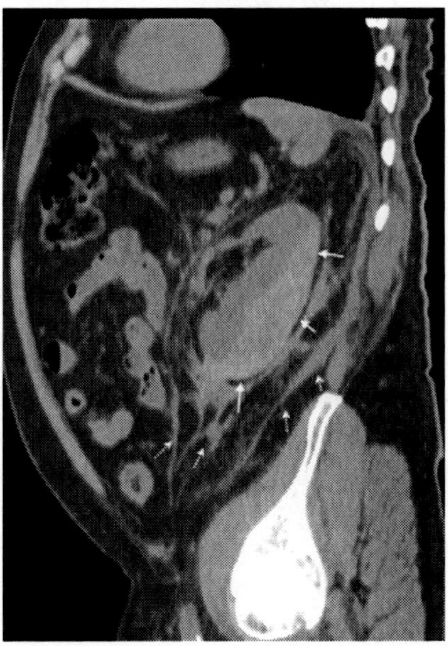

Figure 3. Unenhanced abdominal CT in sagittal view showing a large subcapsular hematoma in the left kidney (solid arrows) and para-renal retroperitoneal hemorrhage (dotted arrows).

On admission his vital signs were entirely normal. Left loin and left upper quadrant tenderness was found. CT revealed a large (mostly subcapsular) hematoma around the single left kidney and a small amount of sanguinous fluid in the peri-renal and left retroperitoneal space (Figure 3). He remained stable and was discharged home after ten days without further misadventure.

## DISCUSSION

Our first patient was admitted first to the department of medicine; the second and third were diagnosed in the emergency department. In all cases there was a considerable diagnostic delay - in the first case, because the diagnosis was not considered, and in the remaining cases - because the patients remained at home (or got up and went home) after their fall.

When an elderly patient presents to the emergency department physicians following a fall, the physicians' prime concern is usually to rule out either bone fractures which are very common due to concurrent osteoporosis or traumatic brain injury. Other common trauma include hematomas and lacerations which may involve much pain and require suturing but are extenal and obvious to the medical team at first sight. Thus, the clinical examination and imaging are both focused on susceptible bones (vertebrae, hip, forearm and hand, leg and ankle, pelvis) and on the patient's neurological condition and the brain. However, the fact that during a fall, relatively minor blunt abdominal or back trauma can cause substantial damage to internal abdominal organs, yet trigger few complaints or suggestive signs at first, remains underappreciated and many clinicians may not be aware of its occurrence and spectrum [8, 17].

Our patients highlight the considerable diagnostic challenge and the variety of serious, little-considered consequences of blunt abdominal trauma due to 'minor' ground-level falls (or other non-penetrating ‘minor’ abdominal trauma) in elderly patients (Table).

Case 1 presented with severe internal bleeding due to a ruptured spleen, yet she was admitted to the department of medicine after the usual imaging which, as often occurs, did not include the abdomen. Her symptoms were ascribed to 'intercurrent' urinary tract infection. A steady drop in the hemoglobin was finally noticed on the 4$^{th}$ hospital day and led to the diagnosis and an emergency curative operation.

The spleen is relatively vulnerable to trauma and is the most commonly damaged viscus in patients sustaining blunt abdominal trauma [18]. Splenic rupture can even occur spontaneously, usually affecting diseased spleens and rarely, a normal spleen of a healthy patient [19]. Trivial trauma including a fall, cough or vomiting as a cause of rupture of a normal spleen has been reported [20], and falls among older adults, being so common [1, 2] constitute an important cause of potential splenic rupture which needs to be recognized in a timely fashion. Hemodynamic instability, falling hemoglobin levels, fracture of lower left ribs and left upper quadrant / back tenderness may occur together (as in our patient) or in different combinations supporting the decision for immediate imaging by CT or ultrasound which should be diagnostic. Other typical signs may include Kehr's sign (shoulder pain secondary to diaphragmatic irritation by the hemoperitoneum), as well as signs of peritonitis (guarding, rebound tenderness). On the other hand, although most of the patients who sustain blunt splenic trauma present acutely, up to 15% may present with delayed rupture days to weeks following the abdominal injury [21].

Our second patient was not even brought to the hospital after she fell at home, her first and also her last fall, since it was ultimately fatal. As identified in the CT scan and confirmed at surgery, her diseased gallbladder ruptured into the colon after the blunt minor trauma of her fall, discharging a large gallstone which caused mechanical bowel obstruction.

Gallstones are an infrequent cause of mechanical ileus but in patients over age 65 they accounts for no less than a quarter of non-strangulated bowel obstruction, particularly in women [22, 23]. Most of these stones are at least 2.5 cm in size and impact in the narrow ileum. Colonic obstruction is unusual due to its width, but does occur, especially in narrowed segments due to previous diverticulitis [23]. The gallbladder is anatomically well-protected and injury during blunt trauma is rare, identified in only 2.1% of 1449 patients [24]. Most reported patients were involved in motor vehicle accidents and had multiple associated intra-abdominal injuries [24, 25]. Importantly, isolated gallbladder rupture is a rare occurrence and in a review of the English literature only 51 cases were identified ranging in age from 3 to 73 years [26]. Interestingly, even a young healthy man who fell in his bathtub after binge drinking could develop an isolated traumatic gallbladder rupture [27] and another young patient manifested cholecystoduodenalcolonic fistula [28]. Isolated gallbladder rupture after a 'simple' fall in *elderly* patients is extremely rare but well established [29]. A fall on the floor associated with blunt abdominal trauma was sufficient to cause a rupture of a diseased gallbladder. At emergency laparotomy, 2000 ml of liquid blood and clots were removed and free, irregular sharp-edged gallstones were found intraperitoneally [29]. Contrast-enhanced CT is a sensitive method of diagnosis. The treatment of choice after stabilizing the patient is an emergency operation and cholecystectomy.

**Table. The great variability of significant intra-abdominal trauma sustained following ground-level falls in patients over 65 years of age***

| |
|---|
| • Spleen<br>Rupture (e.g., Case 1) |
| • Gallbladder<br>Rupture (possible fistula and gallstone ileus) (e.g., Case 2) |
| • Stomach<br>Laceration |
| • Small intestine<br>Perforation<br>Stenoses |
| • Aorta<br>Dissection<br>Embolization<br>Rupture of an abdominal aortic aneurysm |
| • Kidney<br>Hematoma (e.g., Case 3) |
| • Urinary bladder<br>Rupture (mostly associated with osteoporotic fracture of the ramus pubis) |
| • Ureter<br>Rupture (causing hydronephrosis) |

* Events reported are decidedly rare, mostly isolated case reports.

Our third patient was also unusual since we have not been able to find a previous case of blunt trauma during a ground-level fall in the elderly causing renal contusion, hematoma and macrohematuria. Although "isolated" urinary tract blunt injuries are uncommon [30], osteoporotic pubic ramus fractures following falls in elderly patients are not uncommon [31] and can be rarely complicated by bladder injury [32]. One notable case reported is that of an 86-

year-old lady who had tripped from standing height. Pubic ramus fractures were diagnosed and later, difficult to control pain led to the further identification of sacral insufficiency fractures. She then developed hematuria, urinary incontinence and a marked drop in her hemoglobin. Only then, following a rather typical diagnostic delay, was bladder rupture diagnosed, based on a CT IVU, cystogram and MRI [33]. Another extremely rare report describes a ruptured ureter after a fall (from a bus, not stricly ground-level) of a 75-year-old woman [34].

Thus, our series of 546 falls among community dwelling older persons over one year demonstrated the rarity of serious damage to internal abdominal organs but also captured three individual patients with rather unusual internal adverse outcomes. These patients do not reflect the full potential of intra-abdominal injuries that may occur with ground-level falls in the elderly. A review of the literature revealed that rare as they may be, these type of injuries may present to any practitioner. Their rarity often causes a low index of suspicion and potentially dangerous diagnostic delays. Other notable complications of blunt abdominal trauma during falls in elderly patients have been reported and found in our review of the literature. (Table) They include aortic dissection [35] and atheroembolic disease from abdominal aortic aneurysm causing acute limb ischemia [36]. A single report of apparent rupture of an abdominal aortic aneurysm following ground-level fall proved erroneous, after the patient revealed she had been earlier attacked by her husband, but still constitutes an extreme consequence of non-penetrating relatively 'minor' abdominal trauma [37]. Another intriguing report describes an 82-year-old woman who had an axillofemoral bypass graft and presented two weeks after a simple fall with a pulsating mass on her left side caused by localized rupture of a pseudoaneurysm [38]. Other, non-vascular consequences of falls, have also been reported. When fourteen cases of gastric rupture or laceration after blunt abdominal trauma were investigated, 2/14 turned out to be due to falls in elderly patients [39]. Both involved lacerations and not rupture and had no association with a recent meal (in contrast with the cases of rupture of the stomach). Small-intestinal perforation [40] as well as posttraumatic intestinal stenosis with a delayed presentation after a perforation [41] have also been reported. The spectrum of potential internal complications of simple falls in elderly patients is summarized and presented in the Table. Pancreatic injuries were not found and are probably limited to children who fall from height or involved in bicycle handlebar accidents [42].

Falls from height are considered to be high risk for multisystem injury [43]. However, ground-level falls are often thought of as involving low-energy mechanisms and "benign." A recent study of older adults who were hospitalized after a ground-level fall confirmed the high rates of severe injury, readmissions and increased mortality among these patients [44]. For example, among 1352 patients older than 65 years admitted after a fall, approximately half had an injury severity score (ISS) greater than 15 and only 1:3 went home and remained independent. The 1-year mortality for the whole cohort was 33% [44].

In another study, the mortality in the all elderly patients (older than 70 years) who had ground-level fall was significantly higher than in the nonelderly in one large study (4.4% vs. 1.6%, $p < 0.0001$) due to significantly increased incidence of long bone fractures (54.5%), pelvic fracture (7.6%) and intracranial injury (10.6%) [43]. Our study demonstrates that internal injuries, however rare, are also a contributing factor to the increased mortality following falls in the elderly. These events (Table) are very rare and mostly captured and reported as case reports of a single patient. However, the very high and increasing incidence [45] of falls among the elderly and the frequent failure of physicians to consider the possible implications of blunt abdominal trauma associated with 'simple' falls which may leave few external clues mandates attention. Indeed, the recently reported increase in utilization rate of CT imaging for fall victims older than 55 years examined in a level 1 trauma center (approximately 15% increase in imaging per year from 1996 to 2006) may identify more patients with unsuspected serious internal injury [46] and should be encouraged This is particularly true because intra-abdominal injuries (any injury to intraperitoneal and retroperitoneal organs) following blunt trauma (which is considerably more common than a penetrating trauma) cause a substantial proportion of traumatic deaths [47]. Thus, the recent adoption in some centers of routine, whole-body computed tomography (so called "PAN-SCANNING") [48], may be applicable also to elderly patients who experience ground-level falls and are brought to the hospital [49]. Future studies will add to our knowledge on the utility and cost-effectiveness of this approach in trauma secondary to simple falls in the elderly which may rarely be associated with significant occult injury to internal organs.

## CONCLUSION

In conclusion, our small series collected over 1 year and the review of the literature demonstrate the potential of ostensibly minor blunt abdominal or back trauma during falls in elderly persons to be associated with occult serious injury to intra-abdominal organs.

Rupture of a normal spleen, of a chronically inflamed gallbladder with stones or other structures (urinary bladder, abdominal aorta) or contusion of the kidney may occur and patients' presentation may be delayed and misleading.

Higher index of suspicion towards intra-abdominal organ contusion and potential rupture during 'minor' falls is warranted.

## REFERENCES


[1] Hausdorff JM, Rios RA, Edelber HK. Gait variability and fall risk in community-living older adults: a 1-year prospective study. *Arch. Phys. Med. Rehab.* 2001; 82:1050-6.

[2] Tinetti ME. Clinical practice. Preventing falls in elderly persons. *N. Engl. J. Med.* 2003; 348:42-9.

[3] Nevitt MC, Cummings SR, Hudes ES. Risk factors for injurious falls: a prospective study. *J. Gerontol.* 1991; 46:M164-70.

[4] Koski K, Luukinen H, Laippala P, Kivelä SL. Risk factors for major injurious falls among the home-dwelling elderly by functional abilities. A prospective population-based study. *Gerontology* 1998; 44:232-8.

[5] Sattin RW, Lambert Huber DA, DeVito CA, et al. The incidence of fall injury events among the eldely in a defined population. *Am. J. Epidemiol.* 1990; 131:1028-37.

[6] Tinetti ME, Williams CS. Falls, injuries due to falls, and the risk of admission to a nursing home. *N. Engl. J. Med.* 1997; 337:1279-84.

[7] Soriano TA, DeCherrie LV, Thomas DC. Falls in the community-dwelling older adult: a review for primary-care providers. *Clin. Interv. Aging* 2007; 2:545-54.

[8] Helling TS, Watkins M, Evans LL, Nelson PW, Shook JW, Van Way CW. Low falls: an underappreciated mechanism of injury. *J. Trauma* 1999; 46:453-6.

[9] Tinetti ME, Speechley M, Ginter SF. Risk factors for falls among elderly persons living in the community. *N. Engl. J. Med.* 1988; 319:1701-7.

[10] Nevitt MC, Cummings SR, Kidd S, Black D. Risk factors for recurrent nonsyncopal falls. A prospective study. *JAMA* 1989; 261:2663-8.

[11] Ganz DA, Bao Y, Shekelle PG, Rubenstein LZ. Will my patient fall? *JAMA* 2007; 297:77- 86.

[12] Wu TY, Chie WC, Yang RS, et al. Risk factors for single and recurrent falls: a prospective study of falls in community dwelling seniors without cognitive impairment. *Prev. Med.* 2013; 57:511-7.

[13] Weiner DK, Duncan PW, Chandler J, Studenski SA. Functional reach: a marker of physical fraility. *J. Am. Geriatr. Soc.* 1992; 40:203-7.

[14] Schoene D, Wu SM, Mikolaizak AS, et al. Discriminative ability and predictive validity of the timed up and go test in identifying older people who fall: systematic review and meta-analysis. *J. Am. Geriatr. Soc.* 2013; 61:202-8.

[15] Stone KL, Blackwell TL, Ancoli-Israel S, et al. Sleep disturbances and increased risk of falls in older community-dwelling men: the outcomes of Sleep Disorder in Older Men (MrOS) Study. *J. Am. Geriatr. Soc.* 2014;62:299-305.

[16] Schattner A, Mavor E, Adi M. Unsuspected serious abdominal trauma after falls among community-dwelling older adults. *Quart. J. Med. (Oxford)* 2014; 107:649-53.

[17] Nishijima DK, Simel DL, Wisner DH, Holmes JF. Does this adult patient have a blunt intra-abdominal injury? *JAMA* 2012; 307:1517-27.

[18] Fahat GA, Abdu RA, Vanek VW. Delayed splenic rupture: real or imaginary? *Am. Surg.* 1992; 58:340-5.

[19] Schattner A, Meital A, Mavor E. 'Red flag' syncope: spontaneous splenic rupture. *Am. J. Med.* 2104; 127:501-2

[20] Aubrey-Bassler KA, Sowers N. 613 cases of splenic rupture without risk factors or previously diagnosed disease: a systematic review. *BMC Emerg. Med.* 2012; 12:11.

[21] Sowers N, Aubrey-Bassler FK. Trivial trauma and delayed rupture of a normal spleen: a case report. *J. Med. Case Rep.* 2011; 5:591 (http://www.jmedicalcasereports.com/contents/5/1/591).

[22] Reisner RM, Cohen JR. Gallstone ileus: a review of 1001 reported cases. *Am. Surg.* 1994; 60:441-6.

[23] Clavien PA, Richon J, Burgan S, Rohner A. Gallstone ileus. *Br. J. Surg.* 1990; 77:737-42.

[24] Soderstrom CA, Maekawa K, DuPriest RW Jr, Cowley RA. Gallbladder injuries resulting from blunt abdominal trauma. *Ann. Surg.* 1981; 193:60-6.

[25] Sharma O. Blunt gallbladder injuries: presentation of twenty-two cases with review of the literature. *J. Trauma* 1995; 39:576-80.

[26] Schachter P, Czerniak A, Shemesh E, Avigad I, Lotan G, Wolfstein I. Isolated gallbladder rupture due to blunt abdominal trauma. *HPB Surg.* 1989; 1:359-62.

[27] De Rae J, Lamote J, Delvaux G. Isolated traumatic gallbladder rupture. *Acta Chir. Belg.* 2010; 110:370-5.

[28] Griffith CD, Saunders JH. Cholecystoduodenocolic fistula following blunt abdominal trauma. *Br. J. Surg.* 1982; 69:99-100.

[29] Iwacewicz P, Wojskowicz P, Safiejko K, Barczyk J, Dadan J. Traumatic rupture of the gallbladder after blunt abdominal trauma. *Adv. Med. Sci.* 2007; 52: 294-5.

[30] Bariol SV, Stewart GD, Smith RD, McKeown DW, Tolley DA. An analysis of urinary tract trauma in Scotland: impact on management and resource needs. *Surgeon* 2005; 3:27-30.

[31] Kannus P, Palvanen M, Niemi S, Parkkari J, Jarvinen M. Epidemiology of osteoporotic pelvic fractures in elderly people in Finland: sharp increase in 1970-1997 and alarming projections for the new millennium. *Osteoporos. Int.* 2000; 11:443-8.

[32] Thompson SM, Giles MF. A complicated pelvic fracture in an octogenarian. *Quart. J. Med. (Oxford)* 2012; 105:81-2.

[33] Dotchin C, Colman A, Shanshal Y. Bladder rupture following osteoporotic pubic ramus and sacral insufficiency fractures. *Age Ageing* 2010; 39:511-2.

[34] Cross JJ, Wong V, Irving HC, Howdle PD. Ureteric rupture in an elderly patient following minor trauma: case report. *J. Trauma* 1994; 36:594-6.

[35] Kawano H, Ishizaki M, Koide Y, Toda G, Yano K. Thrombosed Stanford type A dissection of the aorta in an elderly patient following a fall. *Intern. Med.* 2005; 44:603-5.

[36] Nigro G, Giovannacci L, Engelberger S, Van den Berg JC, Rosso R. The challenge of posttraumatic thrombus embolization from abdominal aortic aneurysm causing acute limb ischemia. *J. Vasc. Surg.* 2011; 54:840-3.

[37] Chiriano J, Killeen JD, Molkara AM, Bianchi C, Abou-Zamzam AM. J.r. Rupture of an abdominal aortic aneurysm following nonaccidental blunt abdominal trauma. *Vascular* 2010; 18:303-6.

[38] Mousa AY, Nanjundappa A, Abu-Halimah S, Aburahma AF. Traumatic nonanastomotic pseudoaneurysm of axillofemoral bypass graft: a case report and review of the literature. *Vasc. Endovascular. Surg.* 2013; 47:57-60.

[39] Shinkawa H, Yasuhara H, Naka S, et al. Characteristic features of abdominal organ injuries associated with gastric rupture in blunt abdominal trauma. *Am. J. Surg.* 2004; 187:394-7.

[40] Whiteley GS, Penna LK, Bolton JP. Small intestinal perforation following minor trauma. *Injury* 1992; 23:487-8.

[41] Konobu T, Murao Y, Miyamoto S, et al. Posttraumatic intestinal stenosis presenting as a perforation: report of a case. *Surg. Today* 1999; 29:564-7.

[42] Klin B, Abu-Kishk I, Jeruchimov I, et al. Blunt pancreatic trauma in children. *Surg Today* 2011; 41:946-54.

[43] Spaniolas K, Cheng JD, Gestring ML, et al. Ground level falls are associated with significant mortality in elderly patients. *J. Trauma* 2010; 69:821-5.

[44] Ayoung-Chee P, McIntyre L, Ebel BE, et al. Long-term outcomes of ground-level falls in the elderly. *J. Trauma Acute Care Surg.* 2014; 76:498-503.

[45] Hu G, Baker SP. Recent increases in fatal and non-fatal injury among people aged 65 years and over in the USA. *Inj. Prev.* 2010; 16:26-30.

[46] Roudsari B, Psoter KJ, Fine GC, Jarvik JG. Falls, older adults, and the trend in utilization of CT in a level I trauma center. *Am. J. Roentgenology* 2012; 198:985-91.

[47] Isenhour JL, Marx J. Advances in abdominal trauma. *Emerg. Med. Clin. North Am. 2007*; 25:713-33.

[48] Stengel D, Ottersbach C, Matthes G, et al. Accuracy of single-pass whole-body computed tomography for detection of injuries in patients with major blunt trauma. *CMAJ* 2012; 184:869-76.

[49] Dwyer CR, Scifres AM, Stahlfeld KR, et al. Radiographic assessment of ground-level falls in elderly patients: is the "PAN-SCAN" overdoing it? *Surgery* 2013; 154:816-20.

In: Abdominal Trauma ...
Editor: Louise Santiago
ISBN: 978-1-63483-482-7


*Chapter 5*

# Abdominal Aortic Aneurysms and Periodontitis

***Jun-ichi Suzuki[1,*], MD, PhD and Norio Aoyama[2], DDS, PhD***

[1]Department of Advanced Clinical Science and Therapeutics, The University of Tokyo, Japan
[2]Department of Periodontology, Tokyo Medical and Dental University, Japan

## Abstract

Periodontitis is known to be a risk factor for abdominal aortic aneurysm (AAA). However, the influence of periodontitis on AAA development is to be elucidated. The aim of this article was to review the relationship between periodontal bacterial burden and AAA. We focused on the roles of specific periodontopathic bacteria in AAA, matrix metalloproteinases and toll-like receptors in the pathophysiology in the section of experimental analysis. Furthermore, we showed clinical data of periodontitis in patients with AAA and other cardiovascular diseases. We concluded that periodontal pathogens play a critical role in the AAA development.

* Correspondence to Jun-ichi Suzuki; Department of Advanced Clinical Science and Therapeutics, the University of Tokyo, 7-3-1 Hongo, Bunkyo, Tokyo 113-8655, Japan. Phone, 81-3-5800-9116; Fax, 81-3-5800-9182; E-mail: junichisuzuki-circ@umin.ac.jp.

# 1. Introduction

Abdominal aortic aneurysm (AAA) is a common and life-threatening disorder [1, 2]. In AAA development and progression, inflammation is associated with a disruption of the orderly lamellar structure of the aortic media [3]. Pathological examination demonstrated that inflammatory infiltrates in both the media and adventitia was occasionally observed in human AAA tissue [4, 5]. An increased expression of matrix metalloproteinases (MMPs) has also been observed in human aneurysm tissue specimens [6, 7]. Periodontitis is one of the most common chronic infectious diseases in humans. Pathologically, periodontitis is characterized by gingival inflammation and the loss of periodontal support tissue [8]. Periodontopathic bacteria generate host immunological inflammatory responses, thus resulting in the secretion of cytokines and MMPs [9]. This eventually leads to the extracellular matrix destruction of the periodontal tissues [10]. In patients with periodontitis, several inflammatory markers increase [11], meaning that systemic inflammation can be caused by periodontal infection. Salvi et al. showed that periodontopathic bacteria generated host immunological inflammatory responses, thus resulting in the systemic increase of cytokine and MMP expression [9]. A strong association between dental disease and cardiovascular diseases has been demonstrated [12, 13]. Especially, periodontal disease has been reported to be a significant independent risk factor for cardiovascular disease [14]. Previous studies also revealed a deep relationship between periodontal diseases and AAA [15, 16]. Clinical investigations demonstrated that some periodontal pathogens accelerated the progression of AAA [17], however, the specific influence of each periodontal bacterium on AAA was not investigated. Recently, we demonstrated the pathophysiolocial and epidemiological relationship between specific periodontal pathogens and AAA using experimental [18-20] and clinical studies [21, 22]. This article reviews the association between periodontitis and AAA.

# 2. Porphyromonas Gingivalis Is Highly Affected in Systemic Diseases

It is known that more than 700 bacterial species colonize in the oral cavity [23]. Some of them are implicated in the disease progression [24].

*Porphyromonas gingivalis* (*P. gingivalis*) is a bacterium known to be a highly associated with the chronic periodontitis. It can be detected in up to 85% of the disease sites [25], while it is detected rarely in healthy sites. The presence of *P. gingivalis* in a periodontal pocket can predict periodontal disease progression [26]. A reduction of *P. gingivalis* numbers is associated with a resolution of the disease at the affected site [27, 28]. Experimental investigation showed that the infection of *P. gingivalis* in animal models induced an inflammatory response and periodontal bone loss [29]. This bacterium has a number of virulence factors, such as cysteine proteinases (gingipains), lipopolysaccharide (LPS), capsule and fimbriae [30]. However, the roles of virulence factors are still to be elucidated.

## 3. Experimental Models of Periodontopathic Bacteria Infection and AAA

Recently, we revealed that *P. gingivalis* worsened AAA development in experimental murine AAA models [18]. The model showed that *P. gingivalis* significantly increased the aortic diameter in comparison to the vehicle control mice, while another periodontal bacterium, *A. actinomycetemcomitans* showed no statistical increase. Immunohistochemically, the CD8- and MOMA2-positive cell numbers of *P. gingivalis*-infected mice were significantly higher than control animals. We concluded that *P. gingivalis* could accelerate the progression of experimental AAA [18].

To reveal the pathophysiological mechanism, we focused on MMPs in the animal models. Thus, we used clarithromycin (CAM) to suppress MMP activity. We found that the *P. gingivalis*-injected and CAM-treated mice showed a significant decrease in the aortic diameter in comparison to the mice only injected with *P. gingivalis*. Histopathologically, the samples obtained from the *P. gingivalis*-injected and CAM-treated mice showed less elastic degradation. Moreover, the plasma MMP-2 level of the CAM-treated mice significantly decreased. These findings suggest that MMP-2 is a critical factor for developing bacteria-accelerated AAA [19].

Next, we analyzed the role of toll-like receptors (TLRs) because they are key receptors of virulence factors of many periodontal bacteria. To reveal the mechanism, we used TLR deficient mice on *P. gingivali*-accelerated AAA progression.

We found that the *P. gingivalis*-infected TLR-2 deficinet mice showed a significantly lower rate of aortic diameter increase compared to the *P. gingivalis*-infected wild-type mice.

However, the aortic diameter of the *P. gingivalis*-infected TLR-4 deficient mice statistically increased compared to the *P. gingivalis*-infected wild-type mice. Immunohistochemically, the level of MMP-2 in the aneurysmal samples from wild-type mice were higher than that from TLR-2 deficient mice. These findings demonstrate that *P. gingivalis* could accelerate the progression of experimental AAA through TLR-2 signaling [20].

## 4. Clinical Observation of Periodontitis in AAA Patients

Based on the animal studies, we surveyed the periodontal conditions in patients with AAA. Firstly, we studied 12 AAA patients and age and sex-matched 24 patients with non-AAA cardiovascular patients. We examined the patients' oral condition and the presence of periodontal pathogens, *P. gingivalis, A. actinomycetemcomitans* and *P. intermedia* in oral samples. We revealed that the AAA patients had deeper pocket depth compared to the non-AAA patients.

However, the existence of periodontal bacteria was comparable between the two groups. In this observation, we concluded that periodontitis might further affect aneurysm progression compared to other cardiovascular diseases [21]. Next, we compared the periodontal condition between AAA and arrhythmia patients. We studied 142 patients with tachy-arrhythmia (TA) and 25 patients with AAA. We examined patients' oral condition and the presence of *P. gingivalis, A. actinomycetemcomitans* and *P. intermedia* in the patients' saliva and subgingival plaque. We also measured serum antibody titers against the pathogens using ELISA. We found that the patients with AAA had fewer remaining teeth and deeper pocket depth compared to the TA patients. The existence of each periodontal bacterium in their saliva or subgingival plaque and serum antibody titers was comparable between the two groups. We concluded that periodontitis might have a larger affect on aneurysm progression compared to arrhythmia [22].

In these clinical studies, we revealed that periodontitis had progressed further in AAA patients compared to patients with other cardiovascular disease. The result supports the fact that AAA patients had bad oral and periodontal conditions.

While progressed periodontitis was observed in AAA patients compared to patients with other cardiovascular disease, bacterial existence and serum antibody titers were comparable between the groups. These results may deduce a few possible perspectives. Firstly, the specific bacterial burden that plays a key role in AAA development might be concealed because the mean age of the population was too old to detect the difference. Vlachojannis et al. demonstrated that existence rates of periodontal bacteria generally increased by age [31]. Secondly, other periodontal pathogens may aggravate AAA because Kurihara et al. showed that other periodontopathic bacteria were present in AAA specimens [15].

Therefore, surveillance of broader periodontal pathogens in the aortic wall in patients might be useful to reveal the relationship between periodontitis and AAA development.

In conclusion, AAA may be associated with periodontitis and a specific periodontal pathogen may affect the progression of AAA. Further investigation is needed to reveal the detailed pathophysiology in the relationship between AAA and periodontal pathogens.

## ACKNOWLEDGMENTS

This work was supported by Mitsui Life Social Welfare Foundation, Daiwa Security Health Foundation, Mitsui Sumitomo Marine Welfare Foundation, Institute of Geriatric Dentistry Foundation, Institute of St. Luka Life Science Foundation, Health Welfare Foundation, Taiyo Life Welfare Foundation, the 8020 Foundation, Terumo Science Foundation, Pfizer Health Research Foundation, and General Health Promotion Foundation. We thank Dr. Yuichi Izumi, Dr. Mitsuaki Isobe, Dr. Naho Kobayashi, Dr. Tomoya Hanatani, Dr. Norihiko Ashigaki, Dr. Asuka Sekinishi, Dr. Makoto Kaneko, Dr. Yuka Shiheido, Dr. Hiroki Sato, Dr. Atsuhi Akai, Dr. Chisato Takamura, Dr. Masahito Ogawa, Dr. Hirofumi Zempo, Mr. Ryo Watanabe and Ms. Noriko Tamura for their excellent contributions.

## Disclosures

Conflict of Interest: None declared.

## References

[1] Ernst CB. Abdominal aortic aneurysm. *N Engl J Med* 1993; 328: 1167-1172.

[2] Alcorn HG, Wolfson SK, Jr., Sutton-Tyrrell K, Kuller LH, O'Leary D. Risk factors for abdominal aortic aneurysms in older adults enrolled in The Cardiovascular Health Study. *Arterioscler Thromb Vasc Biol* 1996; 16: 963-970.

[3] Longo GM, Xiong W, Greiner TC, Zhao Y, Fiotti N, Baxter BT. Matrix metalloproteinases 2 and 9 work in concert to produce aortic aneurysms. *J Clin Invest* 2002; 110: 625-632.

[4] Bobryshev YV, Lord RS, Parsson H. Immunophenotypic analysis of the aortic aneurysm wall suggests that vascular dendritic cells are involved in immune responses. *Cardiovasc Surg* 1998; 6: 240-249.

[5] Pearce WH, Koch AE. Cellular components and features of immune response in abdominal aortic aneurysms. *Ann N Y Acad Sci* 1996; 800: 175-185.

[6] Freestone T, Turner RJ, Coady A, Higman DJ, Greenhalgh RM, Powell JT. Inflammation and matrix metalloproteinases in the enlarging abdominal aortic aneurysm. *Arterioscler Thromb Vasc Biol* 1995; 15: 1145-1151.

[7] Davis V, Persidskaia R, Baca-Regen L, Itoh Y, Nagase H, Persidsky Y, Ghorpade A, Baxter BT. Matrix metalloproteinase-2 production and its binding to the matrix are increased in abdominal aortic aneurysms. *Arterioscler Thromb Vasc Biol* 1998; 18: 1625-1633.

[8] Choi BK, Jung JH, Suh HY, Yoo YJ, Cho KS, Chai JK, Kim CK. Activation of matrix metalloproteinase-2 by a novel oral spirochetal species Treponema lecithinolyticum. *J Periodontol* 2001; 72: 1594-1600.

[9] Salvi GE, Lang NP. Host response modulation in the management of periodontal diseases. *J Clin Periodontol* 2005; 32 Suppl 6: 108-129.

[10] Ashley RA. Clinical trials of a matrix metalloproteinase inhibitor in human periodontal disease. SDD Clinical Research Team. *Ann N Y Acad Sci* 1999; 878: 335-346.

[11] Reis C, DA Costa AV, Guimarães JT, Tuna D, Braga AC, Pacheco JJ, Arosa FA, Salazar F, Cardoso EM. Clinical improvement following therapy for periodontitis: Association with a decrease in IL-1 and IL-6. *Exp Ther Med* 2014; 8: 323-327.

[12] Mattila KJ, Nieminen MS, Valtonen VV, Rasi VP, Kesäniemi YA, Syrjälä SL, Jungell PS, Isoluoma M, Hietaniemi K, Jokinen MJ. Association between dental health and acute myocardial infarction. *BMJ* 1989; 298: 779-781.

[13] Sakurai K, Wang D, Suzuki J, Umeda M, Nagasawa T, Izumi Y, Ishikawa I, Isobe M. High incidence of actinobacillus actinomycetemcomitans infection in acute coronary syndrome. *Int Heart J* 2007; 48: 663-675.

[14] Mendez MV, Scott T, LaMorte W, Vokonas P, Menzoian JO, Garcia R. An association between periodontal disease and peripheral vascular disease. *Am J Surg* 1998; 176: 153-157.

[15] Kurihara N, Inoue Y, Iwai T, Umeda M, Huang Y, Ishikawa I. Detection and localization of periodontopathic bacteria in abdominal aortic aneurysms. *Eur J Vasc Endovasc Surg* 2004; 28: 553-558.

[16] Paraskevas KI, Mikhailidis DP, Giannoukas AD. Periodontitis and abdominal aortic aneurysms: a random association or a pathogenetic link? *Int Angiol* 2009; 28: 431-433.

[17] Delbosc S, Alsac JM, Journe C, Louedec L, Castier Y, Bonnaure-Mallet M, Ruimy R, Rossignol P, Bouchard P, Michel JB, Meilhac O. Porphyromonas gingivalis participates in pathogenesis of human abdominal aortic aneurysm by neutrophil activation. Proof of concept in rats. *PLoS One* 2011; 6: e18679.

[18] Aoyama N, Suzuki J, Wang D, Ogawa M, Kobayashi N, Hanatani T, Takeuchi Y, Izumi Y, Isobe M. Porphyromonas gingivalis promotes murine abdominal aortic aneurysms via matrix metalloproteinase-2 induction. J Periodontal Res. 2011; 46: 176-183.

[19] Aoyama N, Suzuki J, Ogawa M, Watanabe R, Kobayashi N, Hanatani T, Yoshida A, Ashigaki N, Izumi Y, Isobe M. Clarithromycin suppresses the periodontal bacteria-accelerated abdominal aortic aneurysms in mice. *J Periodontal Res* 2012; 47: 463-469.

[20] Aoyama N, Suzuki J, Ogawa M, Watanabe R, Kobayashi N, Hanatani T, Ashigaki N, Sekinishi A, Izumi Y, Isobe M. Toll-like receptor-2 plays a fundamental role in periodontal bacteria-accelerated abdominal aortic aneurysms. *Circ J* 2013; 77: 1565-1573.

[21] Suzuki J, Aoyama N, Aoki M, Tada Y, Wakayama K, Akazawa H, Shigematsu K, Hoshina K, Izumi Y, Komuro I, Miyata T, Hirata Y, Isobe M. High incidence of periodontitis in Japanese patients with abdominal aortic aneurysm. *Int Heart J* 2014; 55: 268-270.

[22] Suzuki J, Aoyama N, Aoki M, Tada Y, Wakayama K, Akazawa H, Shigematsu K, Hoshina K, Izumi Y, Komuro I, Miyata T, Hirata Y, Isobe M. Incidence of periodontitis in Japanese patients with cardiovascular diseases -A comparison between abdominal aortic aneurysm and arrhythmia. *Heart Vessels* 2014 Apr 16. [Epub ahead of print]

[23] Aas JA, Paster BJ, Stokes LN, Olsen I, Dewhirst FE. Defining the normal bacterial flora of the oral cavity. *J Clin Microbiol* 2005; 43: 5721–5732.

[24] Paster BJ, Olsen I, Aas JA, Dewhirst FE. The breadth of bacterial diversity in the human periodontal pocket and other oral sites. *Periodontology 2000* 2005; 42: 80–87.

[25] Yang HW, Huang YF, Chou MY. Occurrence of Porphyromonas gingivalis and Tannerella forsythensis in periodontally diseased and healthy subjects. *J Periodontol* 2004; 75: 1077–1083.

[26] van Winkelhoff AJ, Loos BG, van der Reijden WA, van der Velden U. Porphyromonas gingivalis, Bacteroides forsythus and other putative periodontal pathogens in subjects with and without periodontal destruction. *J Clin Periodontol* 2002; 29: 1023–1028.

[27] Haffajee AD, Cugini MA, Dibart S, Smith C, Kent RL Jr, Socransky SS. The effect of SRP on the clinical and microbiological parameters of periodontal diseases. *J Clin Periodontol* 1997; 24: 324–334.

[28] Fujise O, Hamachi T, Inoue K, Miura M, Maeda K. Microbiological markers for prediction and assessment of treatment outcome following non-surgical periodontal therapy. *J Periodontol* 2002; 73: 1253–1259.

[29] Hajishengallis G, Liang S, Payne MA Hashim A, Jotwani R, Eskan MA, McIntosh ML, Alsam A, Kirkwood KL, Lambris JD, Darveau RP, Curtis MA.. Low-abundance biofilm species orchestrates inflammatory periodontal disease through the commensal microbiota and complement. *Cell Host Microbe* 2011; 10: 497–506.

[30] Lamont RJ, Jenkinson HF. Life below the gum line: pathogenic mechanisms of Porphyromonas gingivalis. *Microbiol Mol Biol Rev* 1998; 62: 1244–1263.

[31] Vlachojannis C, Dye BA, Herrera-Abreu M, Pikdöken L, Lerche-Sehm J, Pretzl B, Celenti R, Papapanou PN. Determinants of serum IgG responses to periodontal bacteria in a nationally representative sample of US adults. *J Clin Periodontol* 2010; 37: 685-696.

# INDEX

## B



## C

## D



## E

## F



## G

## H



## I

## T

## U



## V



## W



## Y